Workbook for

ESSENTIALS OF HUMAN DISEASES AND CONDITIONS

Seventh Edition

K. Minchella, PhD, CMA (AAMA)

Margaret Schell Frazier, RN, BS, CMA (AAMA)

Retired
Former Chair, Health and Human Services Division
Program Chair, Medical Assisting Program
Ivy Tech State College, Northeast
Fort Wayne, Indiana
Clinical Director
Faith Community Health Clinic
Angola, Indiana
Presently
President/Consultant/Author, M & M Consulting
Hudson, Indiana

Tracie Fuqua, BS, CMA (AAMA)
Medical Assistant Program Chair
Wallace State Community College
Hanceville, Alabama

ELSEVIER

Elsevier
3251 Riverport Lane
St. Louis, Missouri 63043

Content Strategist: Kristin R. Wilhelm
Content Development Specialist: Rebecca Leenhouts
Publishing Services Manager: Deepthi Unni
Project Manager: Srividhya Vidhyashankar

Printed in United States of America

Last digit is the print number: 9 8 7 6 5 4 3 2 1

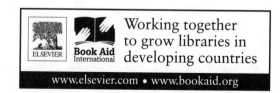

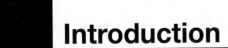

Introduction

Developing an understanding of disease processes is an exciting and fascinating facet of the health care provider's education. Considering that disease conditions are universally experienced, not only do most of us have a natural curiosity about them, but as health care providers, it is essential that we are cognizant of the many components of disease. The study of current medical information on the more common clinical disorders encountered in the health care field presents a challenge to any student.

Essentials of Human Diseases and Conditions, seventh edition, attempts to condense and simplify current medical information on the more common clinical disorders encountered in the health field and physician's office. This companion workbook is intended to present an orderly and concise review of information and to assist you in investigating diseases of the human body. The authors of this workbook, all medical-assisting educators and CMAs-AAMAs, recognize how essential it is for you to have an organized means of reinforcing and reviewing information presented in the text and during class sessions. It is our goal to provide a tool that will bolster the educational experience as you study pathophysiology, as well as to help you approach learning the basics of the human pathologic condition.

Students have previously expressed their desire to have a workbook or study guide to help with studying notes and preparing for examinations. This workbook is a means to review pertinent information, making it more likely that you will remember diseases along with their signs, symptoms, and treatments.

This workbook has been planned to follow the textbook chapters in an orderly fashion. Each chapter of the workbook follows the body systems and presents the review material in the following order:

- Word Definitions
- Glossary Terms
- Short Answer
- Fill-in-the-Blank
- Anatomical Structures
- Patient Screening
- Patient Teaching
- Pharmacology Questions
- Essay Questions
- Certification Exam Review (Multiple Choice)

WORD DEFINITIONS

The sections titled Word Definitions list essential words to help you develop and understand disease entities. The use of a medical dictionary or medical terminology book may be necessary to arrive at the correct meaning of each word as it is used in the textbook.

GLOSSARY TERMS

Glossary terms are boldfaced and/or italicized in each chapter and presented in the glossary section in the back of the textbook (Unless the word is adequately explained in the text adjacent to it's mention). It is suggested that you attempt to recall the information presented in class lecture and then confirm the definition with the textbook glossary.

SHORT ANSWER

Short-answer questions are included in each chapter as a method of providing you with a means of recall. These questions address pertinent facts of selected diseases discussed in the chapter.

FILL-IN-THE-BLANK

Fill-in-the-blank questions provide an opportunity for you to apply one-word or short answers, again to help reinforce and review the information presented. Answers are provided in word lists for rapid recognition.

ANATOMICAL STRUCTURES

Illustrations of anatomical structures and processes are included for labeling. Knowledge of anatomy is crucial to understanding the concepts of disease processes. These labeling exercises are intended to enhance learning.

PATIENT SCREENING

Selected patient-screening scenarios are presented to enable you to relate how you would handle telephone calls to the medical office. For these exercises, you should apply the following general guidelines for patient screening in combination with critical thinking skills to formulate a typical screening response. Five typical phone calls are presented per chapter.

Guidelines for Patient-Screening Exercises

Typically, the medical assistant has the responsibility of screening telephone calls from patients requesting an appointment or reporting treatment progress or lack of progress. The medical assistant is often the initial contact for the patient or patient's family, and critical thinking and a prompt response are required. Many offices have established guidelines regarding the extent of assessment that can be made over the telephone in compliance with state practice acts. It is essential that office staff be aware of and follow office guidelines. Additionally, the medical assistant who is answering the phone may have a list of questions that he or she is expected to ask along with suggestions for appropriate responses regarding appointments or acceptable referrals. Important guidelines for life-threatening situations are listed in the textbook and in this workbook.

It is recommended that you review the information in the text regarding patient screening. The guidelines listed are not intended for diagnosing a caller's medical condition or for providing curative advice. These exercises offer general clues to enable you to recognize the urgency for an appointment, to identify individuals reporting an emergency, and to discern the kind of calls that require referral to the physician for response. These exercises are not intended to focus on the skill of medical triage, which state practice acts generally reserve for certain licensed professionals. When a patient calls, careful listening is essential because the caller often relays information that will help the medical assistant to decide the appropriate action required. Ideally, the outcome of telephone communication between caller and screener will benefit the patient and avoid potential medical and legal problems. Sensitivity to human suffering, strict confidentiality, and a keen awareness of the priority of meeting the needs of patients are necessary skills of the telephone screener and cannot be overstated. The medical assistant must always keep in mind the following important facts listed below.

- Only physicians and nurse practitioners may diagnose disease and prescribe medications.
- Established office protocol must always be followed during the screening process.
- All calls and referrals must be documented according to office policy.
  The following list of serious and life-threatening conditions require immediate assessment and intervention:
- Sudden onset of unexplained shortness of breath
- Crushing pain across the center of the chest
- Difficulty breathing occurring suddenly and rapidly worsening, often in the middle of the night
- Vomiting bright red or very dark "coffee-grounds"-appearing blood
- Sudden onset of weakness and unsteadiness or severe dizziness
- Sudden loss of consciousness or paralysis
- Flashes of light in field of vision
- Sudden and progressively worsening abdominal, flank, or pelvic pain
- Sudden onset of blurred vision accompanied by severe throbbing in the eye
- Children and other individuals with a history of asthma and sudden onset of difficulty breathing
  Additional symptoms requiring prompt assessment include but are not limited to
- Sudden or recent onset of unexplained bleeding including blood in urine, stool, or emesis
- Coughing or spitting up blood
- Unusual and unexplained or heavy vaginal bleeding
- Elevated body temperature of sudden onset or for a prolonged period
- Continued abdominal, back, or pelvic pain
- Sudden onset of headache-type pain
- Children with elevated temperatures or continued vomiting
- Infants with sudden onset of projectile vomiting
  It is essential to document all calls according to office policy and to notify the physician in an emergency situation.

PATIENT TEACHING

Selected patient-teaching scenarios are included to enable you to convey how you would handle patient-teaching opportunities in the medical office. For these exercises, you should apply the following general guidelines for patient teaching.

iv

Introduction

Guidelines for Patient-Teaching Exercises

These exercises are intended to provide you with an opportunity to develop patient-teaching skills. The actual implementation of these skills is dependent on state practice acts and office policies. You have the responsibility to make yourself aware of your state's practice acts and office policy before attempting actual patient teaching. Once you have ascertained that patient teaching is within your scope of practice, you should check office policy for suggested protocol. Many offices have established guidelines for patient teaching, as well as printed materials to assist the health care professional in patient-teaching responsibilities.

- Most offices have patient instructions that are written on the encounter form at the end of the physician's contact with the patient.
- As the patient signs out or before he or she leaves the examination room, the medical assistant reviews these instructions with the patient.
- Often the scheduling of a return visit is the only instruction the physician may write.

Other identified instructions may be the scheduling of additional testing or the inclusion of information about diets or prescribed medications. Although these instructions are a form of patient teaching, reinforcing patient instructions and obtaining patient feedback that confirms his or her understanding of the instructional material is usually considered an essential responsibility for any health care provider. You are encouraged to review general principles of patient teaching as provided in the text.

- It is important to remember that the patient is a partner in health care and that patient teaching, as an ongoing process, requires interaction with the patient and his or her family or caregiver.
- Presenting the material to the patient must be done at the patient's level of understanding.

As you approach each patient-teaching experience, you should have a goal in mind. Usually patients will express goals for a recovery or improvement in their health situation during the intake assessment procedure. Encouraging input from the patient and family or caregiver in setting goals and delegating responsibility for suggested procedures or activities is in the best interest of the patient. The development of a trusting relationship and effective communication helps because individuals are encouraged to assume responsibility for their health and recovery.

The patient-teaching scenarios provided are possible patient-teaching opportunities for the health care professional. The scenarios are presented for every chapter except Chapter 1. You should describe how you would approach the appropriate teaching activity for each situation. Certain patient-teaching opportunities could be duplicated because many teaching concepts are generalized for similar conditions. Once wound care has been explained, it is not necessary for you to repeat this type of instruction in a detailed manner in similar scenarios. Daily weights and requirements for taking medications at the same time every day are examples of patient-teaching opportunities that apply to many patient-teaching situations. Handwashing reminders are an important factor to be mentioned in most teaching opportunities.

PHARMACOLOGY REVIEW QUESTIONS

These questions review pharmacology associated with treatment of diseases and conditions presented within each chapter. The exercises provide a means of identifying types of medication or therapies that are used to treat a patient in certain circumstances.

ESSAY QUESTIONS

One essay question is included for each chapter. These questions will provide you with an opportunity to discuss or explain in detail certain disease-related topics presented in the chapter.

CERTIFICATION EXAMINATION REVIEW

Multiple choice–style questions simulate the typical format found in the certification examination. These questions are incorporated to prepare students for what they will encounter in the certification examination.

It is our goal to furnish you with the optimal study instruments to achieve an understanding of the disease entities you may encounter in a physician's office. We wish you success in your endeavor.

K.Minchella, PhD, CMA (AAMA)
Margaret Schell Frazier, RN, BS, CMA (AAMA)
Tracie Fuqua, BS, CMA (AAMA)

Contents

1 Mechanisms of Disease, Diagnosis, and Treatment

WORD DEFINITIONS

Define the following basic medical terms.

1. Adipose _____

2. Alopecia _____

3. Analgesic _____

4. Cognitive _____

5. Dysfunction _____

6. Ectopic _____

7. Endometrial _____

8. Genetic _____

9. Hematopoietic _____

10. Hypervitaminosis _____

11. Nosocomial _____

12. Palliative _____

13. Preoperatively _____

14. Reflexology _____

15. Systemic _____

16. Transcutaneous _____

17. Transient _____

18. Urticaria _____

19. Visceral _____

20. Differential _____

GLOSSARY TERMS

Define the following chapter glossary terms.

1. Allergen _____

2. Antigen _____

3. Auscultation _____

4. Biopsy _____

5. Cachexia _____

6. Carcinogens _____

7. Dermatome _____

8. Homeostasis _____

9. Karyotype _____

10. Metastasis _____

11. Mutation _____

12. Neoplasm _____

13. Nociceptor _____

14. Pathogenesis _____

15. Phagocytic _____

SHORT ANSWER

Answer the following questions.

1. List the "signs" of disease.

   _____

   _____

2. Diseases that result from an abnormality in or a mutation of a gene are termed what type of disease?

   _____

3. Name tumors that are usually encapsulated and do not infiltrate surrounding tissues.

   _____

   _____

4. Name tumors with invasive cells that multiply excessively and infiltrate other tissues that can represent a serious threat to the patient.

_____

_____

5. Identify the hormone that may be elevated when a patient has prostate cancer.

_____

6. Cite the 2014 statistics for the highest male and female new cancer cases and deaths in the United States as estimated by the American Cancer Society.

_____

7. Any substance that causes an allergic response in a patient is called what?

_____

8. Identify the concept of care that is focused on family support and comfort during life-threatening illness.

_____

9. What does MRSA stand for?

_____

10. What may be the cause of immunodeficiency disorders?

_____

11. What is the single greatest avoidable cause of death and disease?

_____

12. What information from the medical history of a patient is valuable in helping a health care provider assess a patient's condition?

_____

_____

13. What may the physician order to assist with the diagnosis of a patient?

_____

14. Scientists study stem cells to investigate their potential to repair damaged tissue in a field called what?

_____

_____

15. List some examples of predisposing factors related to lifestyle.

_____

_____

16. What are *Staphylococcus* and *Streptococcus*?

_____

17. Identify two environmental factors that may place a patient at increased risk for illnesses, such as pulmonary disease and cancer.

_____

_____

18. Name the type of pain that is usually less severe and has a duration of longer than 6 months. (Inflammatory conditions, such as arthritis and bursitis, are examples.)

_____

19. Name the classification of pain that usually has a sudden onset and is severe in intensity.

_____

20. Name the basic units of heredity that are a small part of a DNA molecule and are located on chromosomes.

_____

21. Are any genetic mutations compatible with life?

_____

22. What are the general treatment options for cancer?

_____

_____

23. Fever, headache, body aches, weakness, fatigue, loss of appetite, and delirium are all symptoms of what?

_____

24. What may be recommended when an individual is known to have a contagious disease that can be easily transmitted to others?

_____

25. Identify the simple precaution that is known to help prevent transmission of pathogens from one person to another, especially in hospital and outpatient medical settings.

_____

4

26. Define immunuodeficiency

_____

27. Define pathogenesis

_____

FILL IN THE BLANKS

Fill in the blanks with the correct terms. A word list has been provided.

Word List

I, 23, absorb, alopecia, anemia, anorexia, benign, breakdown, bruising, (CDC), children, cognitive, diarrhea, dust, emotional, enlarged lymph glands, father, feet, fever, fungi, gene, goal, hands, heat, holistic, infertility, inhibiting, injury, malignant, mold, mother, occurrence, pain, physical, pus, redness, red streaks, risk, sex, social, spiritual, swelling, tissue damage, use, vomiting, young adults

1. Preventive health care emphasizes strategies for _____ a disease and avoiding _____ before it happens.

2. The X and Y chromosomes are known as _____ chromosomes.

3. Each person has _____ pairs of chromosomes. One chromosome from each pair is inherited from the _____, and one is inherited from the _____.

4. The cardinal signs of local infection include _____, _____, _____, _____, _____, _____, and _____.

5. The _____ is a government agency responsible for publishing infectious disease reports in the United States after the diseases are reported to local health departments.

6. Tumors can be classified as either _____ or _____.

7. After evaluation, cancerous tissue is assigned a stage number ranging from I to IV, with stage _____ being an earlier-stage tumor, which carries a better prognosis.

8. The _____ of cancer treatment is to eradicate every cancer cell in the body.

9. Chemotherapy involves the use of chemicals to eradicate cancer cells. The most common side effects are _____, _____, _____, _____, _____, _____, and _____.

10. Physical trauma is the most common cause of death in _____ and _____.

11. A few examples of common allergens that are inhaled include _____, _____, and _____.

12. When a person experiences pain, it is a warning sign that _____ is occurring.

13. Cultural diversity is recognized in the _____ realm of medical treatment because health care providers must meet the needs of culturally diverse patients.

14. Reflexology directs its efforts to the massage of the _____ and _____.

15. Genetic counseling is helpful in predicting _____ of _____ of a gene-linked disease in a family.

16. Small stretches of a deoxyribonucleic acid molecule, situated as a particular site on a chromosome, are known as _____.

17. Malnutrition may be the result of a deficient diet or of disease conditions that do not allow the body to a)_____, b)_____, or _____food.

18. Identify the four cognitive needs that constitute humanness from a holistic perspective.
    a._____ b._____ c._____ d._____

PHARMACOLOGY QUESTIONS

Circle the letter of the choice that best completes the statement or answers the question.

1. Which medication issues are a concern for an elderly patient?
   a. Adverse drug reactions.
   b. Substance abuse.
   c. Overmedication.
   d. All of the above.

2. Categories of infectious disease management medications include:
   a. Antibacterials (antibiotics).
   b. Antifungal and antiviral medications.
   c. Anthelmintics.
   d. All of the above.

3. Medications prescribed for pain are termed:
   a. Antipyretics.
   b. Analgesics.
   c. Antibiotics.
   d. Nutritional agents.

4. An epinephrine kit for self-administration may be prescribed for an individual known to have severe:
   a. Pain.
   b. Depression.
   c. Allergies.
   d. Diabetes.

5. Chemotherapy for cancer involves use of medicines to:
   a. Cause metastasis.
   b. Inhibit an immune response.
   c. Destroy cancer cells.
   d. All of the above.

ESSAY QUESTIONS

Write a response to the following question or statement. Use a separate sheet of paper if more space is needed.

1. Discuss the importance of recognizing cultural diversity in patients.

_____

_____

_____

_____

_____

_____

_____

_____

_____

_____

_____

_____

_____

2. Discuss the immediate and long-term health consequences of exposure to cigarette smoke.

_____

_____

_____

_____

_____

_____

_____

_____

_____

_____

_____

_____

3. Why is MRSA a serious health risk to the community?

_____

_____

_____

_____

_____

_____

_____

_____

_____

_____

_____

_____

4. Describe the difference between signs and symptoms of disease.

_____

_____

_____

5. What is the difference between *staging* and *grading* of tumors?

_____

_____

_____

_____

_____

6. Why is pain necessary?

_____

_____

_____

_____

7. Give an example of alternative therapy

_____

_____

_____

8. Select one of the alternative medicine applications and discuss the experience you or someone you know had using it.

_____

_____

_____

Circle the letter of the choice that best completes the statement or answers the question.

1. An abnormality in or mutation of a gene may produce which of the following?

    a. Inflammatory diseases

    b. Immunodeficiency disorders

    c. Genetic diseases

    d. None of the above

2. What types of tumors tend to metastasize and may spread to distant sites in the body?

    a. Malignant tumors

    b. Benign tumors

    c. Adipose tumors

    d. All of the above

3. Which the following is(are) included in the body's natural defense system against infection?

    a. Mechanical and chemical barriers

    b. Inflammatory response

    c. Immune response

    d. All of the above

4. Which statement describes how a pathogen can cause disease?

    a. By releasing harmful toxins into the body

    b. Invasion and destruction of living tissue

    c. Infiltration of dead tissue

    d. Both a and b

5. Systemic manifestations of severe allergic responses include:

    a. Arthralgia.

    b. Status asthmaticus.

    c. Anaphylaxis.

    d. All of the above.

6. Which concept of medical care focuses on the needs of the whole person—spiritual, cognitive, social, physical, and emotional?

    a. Holistic

    b. Hospice

    c. Osteopathy

    d. None of the above.

7. The concept of care that affirms life and neither hastens nor postpones death is the:

    a. Holistic.

    b. Hospice philosophy.

    c. Osteopathy.

    d. None of the above.

8. Which of the following is responsible for stimulating the immune system to produce antibodies?

    a. Mutation

    b. Chromosome

    c. Antigen

    d. None of the above

9. A new tissue growth or a tumor is called a:

    a. Mutation.

    b. Neoplasm.

    c. Biopsy.

    d. None of the above.

10. Which predisposing factors are related to a person's lifestyle?

    a. Gender

    b. Age

    c. Pollution of air and water

    d. Smoking, poor nutrition, lack of exercise, and risky sexual behavior

11. Pain as described by the patient is:

    a. Objective.

    b. Experienced the same in everyone.

    c. Subjective and individualized.

    d. Never referred to other regions of the body.

12. Patient education:

    a. Helps improve patient and family coping.

    b. Is interactive.

    c. Is based on the patient's plan of care.

    d. All of the above.

13. The tumor Gleason grade reflects:

    a. The stage of the tumor.

    b. The degree of abnormal microscopic appearance of the tumor cells.

    c. The location of the tumor.

    d. None of the above.

14. The TNM system of staging a malignant tumor assesses for:

    a. Tumor size.

    b. The extent of lymph node involvement.

    c. The number of distant metastases.

    d. All of the above.

15. Aging is a risk factor for the onset of many health issues, including:

    a. More stress.

    b. Adverse drug reactions.

    c. Immunosenescence.

    d. All of the above.

Scenario

Scenario will provide students to use critical thinking skills to determine the various possible answer. Some research may be necessary to include an evidence-based answer.

1. As the American population over the age of 65 continues to increase, so do the life stressors such as financial hardships, loss of loved ones, onset of chronic diseases, and potential drug therapy misuse. These factors and other contribute to how the aging patients might comply with treatments.

    A. Describe supportive measures that medical staff could offer to help reduce financial hardships for the aging population.

    _____

    _____

    _____

    _____

    _____

    B. Discussion compliance strategies to ensure proper medical treatment for the aging patient.

    _____

    _____

    _____

    _____

    _____

2 Developmental, Congenital, and Childhood Diseases and Disorders

WORD DEFINITIONS

Define the following basic medical terms.

1. Acyanotic _____

2. Amniocentesis _____

3. Adduction _____

4. Anencephaly _____

5. Apnea _____

6. Arthritis _____

7. Ataxic _____

8. Bicornate _____

9. Bursitis _____

10. Congenital _____

11. Dystrophy _____

12. Foramen ovale _____

13. Hydrocephalus _____

14. Hypovolemia _____

15. Lethargy _____

16. Myopia _____

17. Nosocomial _____

18. Palpable _____

19. Posterior _____

20. Postnatal _____

21. Postpartum _____

22. Prenatal _____

23. Tracheostomy _____

24. Transdermal _____

GLOSSARY TERMS

Define the following chapter glossary terms.

1. Anastomosis _____

2. Anorexia _____

3. Antipyretic _____

4. Cyanosis _____

5. Dysphagia _____

6. Dyspnea _____

7. Electromyography _____

8. Hemolysis _____

9. Hypertrophic _____

10. Hypoxia _____

11. Meconium _____

12. Necrosis _____

13. Normal flora _____

14. Patent _____

15. Photophobia _____

16. Phototherapy _____

17. Pruritus _____

18. Stenosis _____

19. Syncope _____

20. Tachycardia _____

21. Tachypnea _____

SHORT ANSWER

Answer the following questions.

1. Which type of congenital disorders can be diagnosed by amniocentesis?

   _____

2. What occurs when there is a failure in the separation process of identical twins before the 13th day after fertilization?

   _____

3. Is the condition of conjoined twins more prevalent in females or males?

   _____

4. What is the weight range for premature infants?

   _____

5. List three causes of prematurity.

   _____

6. Name an example of an abnormality that may be detected by examination of amniotic fluid.

   _____

7. What is another name for infant respiratory distress syndrome (IRDS)?

   _____

8. List symptoms and signs of hypertrophic cardiomyopathy.

   _____

   _____

9. Explain how retinopathy of prematurity (retrolental fibroplasia) is diagnosed.

   _____

   _____

10. List symptoms and signs of Down syndrome.

    _____

11. What is considered to be the most common crippling condition of children?

    _____

12. What is the cause of cerebral palsy?

    _____

13. Identify the most serious form of spina bifida.

_____

14. Surgical intervention for myelomeningocele is recommended when?

_____

15. If a baby is born with anencephaly, what is the prognosis?

_____

16. What are the two forms of Robinow syndrome?

_____

17. Trace fetal circulation from umbilical vein through system to umbilical artery.

_____

18. Describe patent ductus arteriosus.

_____

19. Name the most common congenital cardiac disorder.

_____

20. What color is the skin of a baby born with tetralogy of Fallot?

_____

21. Cite the statistics for the occurrence of cleft abnormalities.

_____

22. List the major clinical manifestations of cystic fibrosis.

_____

23. Name the most common kidney tumor of childhood.

_____

24. List causes of anemia.

_____

25. List examples of helminths that can live in the gastrointestinal tract.

_____

26. Klinefelter's syndrome and Turner's syndrome are both chromosome disorders. Which one affects males, and which one affects females?

_____

27. The test for cystic fibrosis that measures the levels of sodium and chloride is called what?

_____

28. Identify the organism responsible for causing chickenpox.

_____

29. List a few precautions women can take to help decrease the risk of abnormal fetal development.

_____

30. Cite possible causes of nongenetic congenital abnormalities that may be present in a child.

_____

_____

31. List the three major types of cerebral palsy.

_____

_____

_____

32. Explain the goal of treatment for cerebral palsy.

_____

33. List the four abnormalities present in the heart of an infant who has tetralogy of Fallot.

_____

_____

_____

_____

34. What are some of the physical characteristics that a child with Down syndrome will exhibit?

_____

_____

35. Explain the treatment measures that may be used if clubfoot is present.

_____

_____

36. What treatment options are available to a baby born with patent ductus arteriosus (PDA)?

_____

_____

17

Chapter **2**   **Developmental, Congenital, and Childhood Diseases and Disorders**

37. Define phimosis.

_____

38. List the symptoms associated with adenoid hyperplasia.

_____

39. What is the method of transmission for lead poisoning?

_____

40. Discuss possible causes and prevention of SIDS.

_____

41. Distinguish between croup and epiglottitis.

_____

42. Define an autosomal inherited condition

_____

FILL IN THE BLANKS

Fill in the blanks with the correct terms. A word list has been provided.

Word List

3, 8, 21, fifteenth, eighteenth, airborne, brain damage, cardiac, cyanosis, diphtheria toxoid, droplet, dyspnea, electromyography (EMG), elevated serum creatinine kinase (CK), environmental, erythromycin, folic acid, genetic, good, great vessels, intellectual developmental disorder, mewing, muscle biopsy, one vein, pneumonia, pyloric stenosis, respiratory syncytial virus (RSV), shunt, small, syncope, two arteries, vitamin A, viruses

1. The diagnosis of congenital anomalies in a fetus can be accomplished by amniocentesis between the
   _____ and _____ week of pregnancy.

2. An infant with bronchopulmonary dysplasia (BPD) is very susceptible to respiratory infections, such as
   _____ and _____.

3. Muscular dystrophy is diagnosed by _____, _____, and _____.

4. The exact cause of spina bifida is unknown. However, _____ and _____ factors may play a role.
   In addition, a decrease in the amount of _____ and _____ may contribute to the occurrence.

5. Treatment for hydrocephalus usually includes placing a(an) _____ in the ventricular or subarachnoid
   spaces to drain off the excessive cerebrospinal fluid (CSF).

6. An infant with cri du chat syndrome exhibits an abnormally _____ head; and, if born alive, the infant will
   have a weak _____, mewing cry.

7. The umbilical cord contains _____ and _____.

8. Congenital _____ defects are developmental anomalies of the heart or _____ of the heart.

9. An atrial septic defect that is large would cause pronounced symptoms of _____, _____,
   and _____.

18

10. The prognosis for cleft lip and cleft palate is _____ with surgical repair.

11. An infant with _____ _____ has episodes of projectile vomiting after feedings. The onset of symptoms usually begins within 2 to 3 weeks after birth.

12. Phenylketonuria is an inborn error in the metabolism of amino acids that causes _____ and _____ if not treated.

13. Diphtheria can be prevented by the administration of _____ to produce active immunity.

14. The causative agent of mumps is a(an) _____ virus, which is spread by _____ nuclei from the respiratory tract.

15. The drug of choice to treat pertussis (whooping cough) is _____.

16. A common disease in infancy, bronchiolitis is usually caused by a(an) _____.

17. The incubation period for tetanus is _____ to _____ days, with onset commonly occurring at about _____ days.

Chapter 2 Developmental, Congenital, and Childhood Diseases and Disorders

ANATOMIC STRUCTURES

Label the following anatomic diagrams. For number 2, identify the correct heart defect that each diagram illustrates.

1. Circulation patterns before and after birth

Fetal Circulation

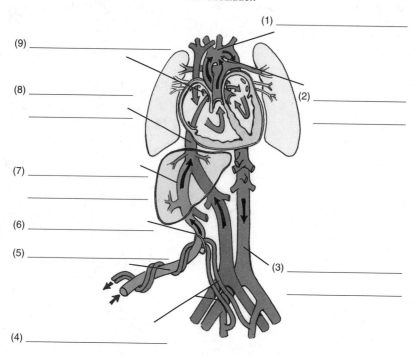

(1) _____

(9) _____

(8) _____

_____

(2) _____

_____

(7) _____

_____

(6) _____

(5) _____

(3) _____

_____

(4) _____

Circulation after Birth

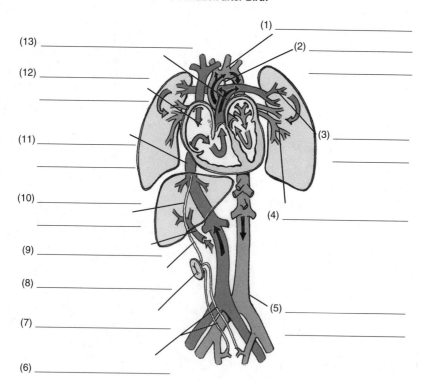

(1) _____

(13) _____

(2) _____

(12) _____

_____

_____

(3) _____

(11) _____

_____

(10) _____

_____

(4) _____

(9) _____

(8) _____

(5) _____

(7) _____

_____

(6) _____

2. Heart defects

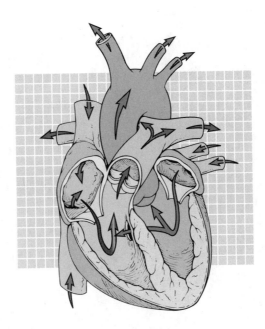

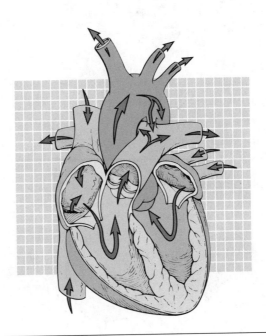

Chapter **2** **Developmental, Congenital, and Childhood Diseases and Disorders**

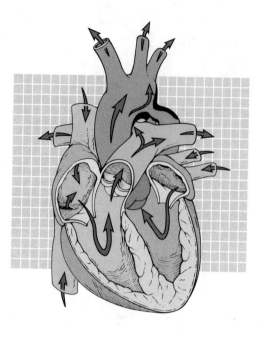

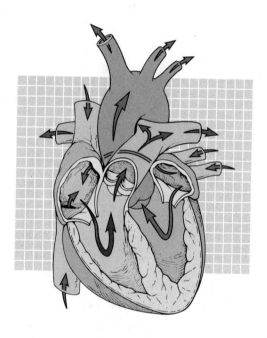

Chapter **2** **Developmental, Congenital, and Childhood Diseases and Disorders**

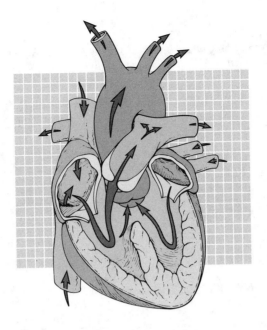

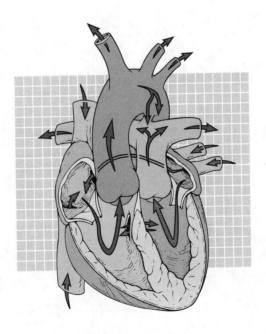

PATIENT SCREENING

For each scenario that follows, explain how and why you would schedule an appointment or suggest a referral based on the patient's reported symptoms. First review the "Guidelines for Patient-Screening Exercises" found on p. iv in the Introduction.

1. The mother of a 6-month-old infant calls the office requesting an appointment for her child. She advises that she thinks the child's head appears swollen and that there are areas that appear to be bulging. What is your response regarding the appointment?

   _____

   _____

   _____

2. The mother of a 3-year-old boy calls to report that her child had the onset of vomiting and abdominal pain during the night and is now experiencing blood in his urine. She says that she just noticed a swelling on his left side toward his back. She requests an appointment. What is your response regarding the appointment?

   _____

   _____

   _____

3. The mother of a 15-day-old infant son reports that he started having episodes of vomiting, with the emesis "shooting out of his mouth" after feeding. She also reports that the infant appears hungry, continues to feed, and has not gained any weight. How do you respond to this phone call?

   _____

   _____

   _____

4. Just as the office is closing for the day, a mother calls about her child who just started experiencing signs and symptoms of respiratory distress including hoarseness; fever; a harsh, high-pitched cough; and a funny, high-pitched sound during inspiration. The physician has already left the office for the day. How do you handle this call?

   _____

   _____

   _____

5. A mother calls to report that her three children have been complaining of being fatigued; having headaches; and having stomach, muscle, and joint pain for the past 2 weeks. She also states there has been a significant change in their behavior. How do you handle this call?

   _____

   _____

   _____

6. A father calls the office inquiring about what he should do. His 6-year-old son has just come home from school and he noticed small, reddened areas with tiny blisters on the boy's face, neck, arms, and now chest. He is asking about school attendance for the next day. How would you respond to this father?

_____

_____

_____

7. The mother of a 3-year-old girl calls the office concerned that her daughter is experiencing abdominal pain. On checking her child she has noticed what she thinks is an abdominal mass. She says the skin around the girl's eyes is dark and looks like raccoon eyes. How would you handle this call?

_____

_____

_____

PATIENT TEACHING

For each of the following scenarios, outline the appropriate patient teaching that you would perform. First review the "Guidelines for Patient-Teaching Exercises" found on p. iv in the Introduction.

1. SPINA BIFIDA
   Parents have brought a previously diagnosed child to the office for a routine visit. They missed the last regularly scheduled appointment. During the intake assessment they told you that the child had no problems, so they did not come. How do you handle this parent-teaching opportunity?

   _____

   _____

   _____

2. PYLORIC STENOSIS
   An infant has been seen on his or her first postoperative visit. How do you handle this parent-teaching opportunity?

   _____

   _____

   _____

3. CHICKENPOX
   A child has just been diagnosed with chickenpox. How do you handle this parent-teaching opportunity? Parent again

   _____

   _____

   _____

4. TONSILLITIS

A child has just been diagnosed with tonsillitis. The physician has prescribed a round of antibiotics for the child. He has also made note to the parents to ensure that the child has adequate hydration. How do you handle this parent-teaching opportunity? Parent again

_____

_____

_____

5. ASTHMA

A child has been examined for a severe episode of recurring asthma. The physician has prescribed a prophylactic inhalant to be used before exposure. In addition, the child has a prescription for a bronchodilator medication that he is inconsistent in taking. How do you handle this patient/parent-teaching opportunity? Patient/parent teaching?

_____

_____

_____

PHARMACOLOGY QUESTIONS

Circle the letter of the choice that best completes the statement or answers the question.

1. Closure of patent ductus arteriosus may be attempted by drug therapy using:

   a. Steroid therapy.

   b. An antiprostaglandin.

   c. Digitalis.

   d. An ace inhibitor.

2. Medications that contain _____ may mask the symptoms of Reye's syndrome and are generally avoided in the treatment of chickenpox.

   a. Acetaminophen

   b. Azithromycin

   c. Aspirin

   d. Acyclovir

3. Mumps is a childhood disease that is best prevented by:

   a. The MMR vaccine.

   b. The Gardasil vaccine.

   c. Broad spectrum antibiotics.

   d. Cough medicines.

4. Acute tonsillitis (strep positive) is generally treated with _____ to prevent rheumatic fever or rheumatic heart disease.

   a. Estradiol (Estrace)

   b. Prednisone

   c. Penicillin

   d. Promethazine

5. Roundworms, pinworms, and tapeworm can be treated with which medication?

    a. Melamine (Antivert)

    b. Finasteride (Proscar)

    c. Mebendazole (Vermox)

    d. Medroxyprogesterone (Provera)

6. Childhood asthma can be treated with all of the following except:

    a. Albuterol (Proventil).

    b. Budesonide (Pulmicort).

    c. Tetracycline (Sumycin).

    d. Corticosteroids.

Referring to the CDC Childhood and Adolescent Immunization Schedule in the textbook, answer the following questions.

1. When should an infant receive the first in the series of hepatitis B immunizations?

    _____

2. At what age should a child receive the first varicella immunization?

    _____

3. At what age should a child receive the second MMR?

    _____

4. At what age should a child receive influenza vaccine?

    _____

5. What is the recommended schedule for *Haemophilus influenzae* type B immunizations?

    _____

ESSAY QUESTIONS

Write a response to the following question or statement. Use a separate sheet of paper if more space is needed.

1. Compare the symptoms of the three major types of cerebral palsy: spastic cerebral palsy, athetoid cerebral palsy, and ataxic cerebral palsy.

_____

_____

_____

_____

_____

_____

_____

_____

_____

_____

2. Discuss the implications of children born with fetal alcohol syndrome on family, health care system, and educational system.

_____

_____

_____

_____

_____

_____

_____

_____

_____

_____

_____

3. Contact a Shriner and ask about services provided to children with orthopedic or cranial facial anomalies. Discuss how families may be made aware of the services.

_____

_____

_____

_____

_____

_____

_____

_____

_____

_____

4. Cystic fibrosis is considered to be a fatal disease. Discuss some of the possible feelings of the parents and also of the individual when he/she is old enough to begin to understand the implications of the disease.

_____

_____

_____

_____

_____

_____

_____

_____

_____

_____

29

Chapter **2** **Developmental, Congenital, and Childhood Diseases and Disorders**

5. Discuss possible conversations with parents about the necessity of having their children immunized according to the CDC recommended guidelines.

_____

_____

_____

_____

_____

_____

_____

_____

_____

_____

6. Discuss the necessity of older individuals being current on pertussis immunizations.

_____

_____

_____

_____

_____

_____

_____

_____

_____

_____

7. Compare cyanotic and non-cyanotic congenital cardiac defects.

_____

_____

_____

_____

_____

_____

_____

_____

_____

_____

8. Rubella is a highly contagious viral disease. Explain how it is diagnosed and treated.

_____

_____

_____

_____

_____

9. What is the difference between prognosis and diagnosis in Hypertrophic Cardiomyopathy?

_____

_____

_____

_____

_____

10. When an anomaly such as cleft lip and palate is found during newborn examination, h ow should patient screening be conducted?

_____

_____

_____

_____

11. There has been rapid increase of contagious diseases in the United States, measles and mumps. Explain two of the most significant reasons for these increases.

_____

_____

_____

_____

12. Describe the symptoms and signs of blood disorders.

_____

_____

_____

_____

CERTIFICATION EXAMINATION REVIEW

Circle the letter of the choice that best completes the statement or answers the question.

1. Reye's syndrome has been associated with the use of:

   a. Acetaminophen.

   b. Ibuprofen.

   c. Aspirin.

   d. All of the above.

2. Loss of appetite, vomiting, irritability, and ataxic gait are symptoms associated with:

   a. Muscular dystrophy.

   b. Anemia.

   c. Lead poisoning.

   d. All of the above.

3. The leading cause of absenteeism in schoolchildren is:

    a. Asthma.

    b. Strep infections.

    c. Bronchitis.

    d. Otitis media.

4. The failure of the testicle(s) to descend into the scrotum is called:

    a. Cryptorchidism.

    b. Testicular torsion.

    c. Phimosis.

    d. Turner's syndrome.

5. If a child is born with tetralogy of Fallot, how many actual heart defects are present?

    a. Two

    b. Three

    c. Four

    d. One

6. When a person is diagnosed with leukemia, there will be a(an):

    a. Increase in white blood cells.

    b. Decrease in white blood cells.

    c. Normal white blood cell count.

    d. Decrease in platelets.

7. Sensitivity to iron or cow's milk may cause:

    a. Cystic fibrosis.

    b. Infantile colic.

    c. Pyloric stenosis.

    d. All of the above.

8. The most progressive form of muscular dystrophy is:

    a. Occulta.

    b. Duchenne's.

    c. Down syndrome.

    d. Myotonic.

9 One way to prevent epidemics of contagious diseases is:

    a. Aspirin.

    b. Immunizations.

    c. Multivitamins.

    d. Cold and cough medications.

10. Hypertension, hematuria, and pain are symptoms of:

    a. Leukemia.

    b. Cystic fibrosis.

    c. Wilms' tumor.

    d. All of the above.

11. The number one cause of death in children between the ages of 1 month and 1 year is:

    a. Sudden infant death syndrome.

    b. Cystic fibrosis.

    c. Down syndrome.

    d. Erythroblastosis fetalis.

12 Rheumatic fever, kidney complications, and rheumatic heart disease may be complications of untreated:

    a. Lead poisoning.

    b. Tonsillitis caused by A beta-hemolytic streptococci.

    c. Vomiting and diarrhea.

    d. Anemia.

13. Intracranial pressure is present when cerebrospinal fluid accumulates in the skull when the patient has:

    a. Hydrocephalus.

    b. Spina bifida.

    c. Fetal alcohol syndrome.

    d. Congenital rubella syndrome.

14. Women of childbearing age are advised to increase their intake of _____ to help prevent neural tube defects in their unborn child.

    a. Iron

    b. Folic acid

    c. Calcium

    d. Vitamin A

15. An electrocardiogram is suggested for athletes to identify those who may have:

    a. Asthma.

    b. Hypertrophic cardiomegaly.

    c. Cerebral palsy.

    d. Rheumatic heart disease.

16. The most common childhood malignancy is:

    a. Leukemia.

    b. Wilms' tumor.

    c. Hirschsprung's disease.

    d. Meningocele.

17. The condition where the foreskin of the penis does not have adequate opening to allow it to be pulled back over the end of the penis is called:

    a. Testicular torsion.

    b. Phimosis.

    c. Cryptorchism.

    d. Wilms' tumor.

18 Erythroblastosis fetalis is a condition caused by:

    a. Iron deficiency.

    b. Rh incompatibility.

    c. Alcohol consumption during pregnancy.

    d. Lead poisoning.

19. Childhood obesity may be caused by:

    a. The child eating too much food and not exercising enough.

    b. Fast-food restaurant type of food.

    c. Snacks, such as cookies, crackers, candy, and sodas that are high in calories.

    d. All of the above.

20. Treatment of hydrocephalus includes:

    a. Starting surgical intervention to insert a shunt.

    b. Closing the opening.

    c. Fusing the skull.

    d. Starting diuretics.

21. Preterm birth or prematurity is the result of birth before which week of gestation?

    a. 30

    b. 35

    c. 37

    d. 40

22. Muscular Dystrophy is a progressive degeneration and weakening of the skeletal muscles abnormally vulnerable to injury. MD initially affects which muscles?

    a. Shoulders, hips, thighs, and calves of the legs.

    b. Fingers, hands, arms and shoulders.

    c. Toe, ankle, knee, and hip joints.

    d. Abdominal, solar plexus, diaphragm and pectoralis

23. Croup is an acute, severe inflammation and obstruction to which of the following?

    a. tonsils

    b. larynx

    c. respiratory tract

    d. small air passages of the lungs

24. Which measures are treatment for lead poisoning?

    a. Antiemetics help to control nausea and vomiting

    b. Eliminating the source of poisoning.

    c. Sedation is given for convulsions.

    d. Induce vomiting.

Scenarios

Scenario 1 Parents bring the newborn baby into the medical facility with questions about their child's condition of Talipes Equinovarus otherwise known as club foot.

QUESTIONS

a. What is wrong with my baby?

_____

_____

_____

_____

b. What causes this?

_____

_____

_____

_____

c. What is meant by the term true club foot?

_____

_____

_____

_____

d. What is the treatment for this condition?

_____

_____

_____

_____

e. What if these methods are unsuccessful?

_____

_____

_____

_____

f. What is the prognosis?

_____

_____

_____

_____

g. What should the parents be taught?

_____

_____

_____

_____

Scenario 2

Parents who are dealing with their newborn infant who has congenital defects suffer from stress, anxiety, fear, and disappointment.

QUESTIONS

a. What can the medical staff do to be supportive of the parents?

_____

_____

_____

_____

b. What community resources are available to share with the parents?

_____

_____

_____

_____

c. Describe how to manage the parent who is repeatedly calling the office for an appointment?

_____

_____

_____

_____

3 Immunologic Diseases and Conditions

WORD DEFINITIONS

Define the following basic medical terms.

1. Allograftc _____

2. Arthralgia _____

3. Conjunctivitis _____

4. Ecchymosis _____

5. Endocrinopathies _____

6. Exacerbate _____

7. Flatulence _____

8. Hypocalcemia _____

9. Lysis _____

10. Neuritis _____

11. Ocular _____

12. Splenomegaly _____

13. Spondylitis _____

14. Stomatitis _____

15. Thyroiditis _____

16. Uveitis _____

17. Vasculitis _____

GLOSSARY TERMS

Define the following chapter glossary terms.

1. Antibodies _____

2. Antigens _____

3. Atrophy _____

4. Autoimmune _____

5. Discoid _____

6. Enzyme-linked immunosorbent assay _____

7. Erythrocyte sedimentation rate _____

8. Idiopathic _____

9. Immunocompetent _____

10. Immunodeficiency _____

11. Immunoglobulins _____

12. Immunosuppressive _____

13. Ischemic _____

14. Macrophages _____

15. Megakaryocytes _____

16. Megaloblastic _____

17. Opportunistic infections _____

18. Petechiae _____

19. Phagocytes _____

20. Phagocytosis _____

21. Reticuloendothelial _____

22. Retrovirus _____

23. Tetany _____

24. Thrombocytopenia _____

25. Western blot test _____

SHORT ANSWER

Answer the following questions.

1. What would be included as primary lymphoid tissues?

_____

2. Which structures are considered the first line of defense against foreign substances or antigens?

_____

3. Name the two types of acquired specific immunity.

_____

_____

4. What is the name of the substance that coats B cells, providing them with the ability to recognize foreign protein, stimulating the antigen-antibody reaction?

_____

5. What is the name of the virus that causes acquired immunodeficiency syndrome (AIDS)?

_____

6. Identify the organism responsible for causing a fungal infection of the mucous membranes of the mouth, genitalia, or skin. It is a common opportunistic infection observed in patients who have AIDS.

_____

7. Is there a cure for AIDS?

_____

8. Severe combined immunodeficiency (SCID) results from disturbances in the development and function of which cells?

_____

9. Identify the treatment option for SCID.

_____

10. When a patient has autoimmune hemolytic anemia, antibodies destroy what?

_____

11. The clinical symptoms of thrombocytopenic purpura (ITP) are due to a deficiency of what element of the blood that assists in blood clotting?

_____

12. What is the name of the fibrous, insoluble protein that is the main component of connective tissue?

_____

13. Systemic lupus erythematosus is frequently referred to as what?

_____

14. Name the disease that causes thickening of the skin.

_____

15. Sjögren's syndrome is more commonly found in families that have which illnesses?

_____

_____

16. Name the most severe form of arthritis that commonly causes deformity and disability.

_____

17. Juvenile rheumatoid arthritis affects children of what ages?

_____

18. Is ankylosing spondylitis (AS) more prevalent in males or females?

_____

19. Name the blood tissue antigen that is present in 90% of individuals who have AS.

_____

20. Cite the body system that is affected when the patient is diagnosed with multiple sclerosis.

_____

21. What is the common characteristic of multiple sclerosis?

_____

22. List examples of organs or tissues that can be transplanted successfully.

_____

_____

23. Explain the difference between active and passive immunity.

_____

_____

24. Discuss the medical management for a patient diagnosed with AIDS.

_____

_____

25. Explain the precautions for immunizing children with Bruton's agammaglobulinemia.

_____

_____

26. What defines immunoincompetence?

_____

_____

27. Explain what the patient with Goodpasture syndrome may experience?

_____

_____

28. Collagen constitutes what percent of the total body protein?

_____

_____

FILL IN THE BLANKS

Fill in the blanks with the correct terms. A word list has been provided. Words used twice are indicated with a (2).

Word List

acute glomerulonephritis, antifungal, autoantibodies, B-cell deficiency, cardiovascular, cells, cold, deformity, eyes, function, HAART, hematuria, hydrochloric acid, idiopathic, immune system (2), immunoglobulins, infections, inflammation, laboratory tests, mouth, muscles, numbness, pinnas, platelets, proteinuria, reduction, renal failure, sore tongue, spinal column, stress, sunlight, thrombocytopenia, tingling, vitamin B_{12}, weakness (2), western blot, IgA, SCID

1. The _____ is responsible for a complex response to the invasion of the body by foreign substances.

2. B cells are coated with _____, giving them the ability to recognize foreign protein and stimulate an antigen-antibody reaction.

3. If a patient has a positive rapid human immunodeficiency virus (HIV) antibody test or a positive enzyme-linked immunosorbent assay for HIV antibodies, the tests should be confirmed with another test called a(an) _____.

4. Common variable immunodeficiency is an acquired _____ that results in an absence of antibody production or function, or both.

5. DiGeorge's anomaly is identified in children who have structural anomalies, such as wide-set, downward-slanting _____; low-set ears with notched _____; a small _____; and _____ defects.

6. The mainstay of treatment for chronic mucocutaneous candidiasis is _____ agents.

7. The child who has the diagnosis of Wiskott-Aldrich syndrome experiences _____ and eczema.

8. Autoimmune diseases occur when _____ develop and begin to destroy the body's own _____.

9. Symptoms associated with pernicious anemia include a _____, _____, _____, and _____ in the extremities. They may also include disturbances in digestion as a result of a decrease in the production of _____.

10. Monthly injections of _____ are used to treat pernicious anemia.

11. The cause of thrombocytopenic purpura is often considered _____, although antibodies that reduce the life of _____ have been found in most cases.

12. Symptoms of Goodpasture's syndrome are _____, relatively acute _____ with _____, anemia, hemoptysis, and _____.

13. Treatment options for collagen diseases are directed at quieting the overactive _____.

14. The primary objectives of treatment for rheumatoid arthritis are _____ of _____ and pain, preservation of joint _____, and prevention of joint _____.

15. The _____ is usually affected by ankylosing spondylitis.

16. The most common symptom of polymyositis is _____ of the _____.

17. Prolonged exposure to _____, _____, _____, and emotional _____ exacerbate the symptoms of myasthenia gravis.

18. Failure to produce adequate levels of _____ is the most common immunologic defect in the general population.

19. Testing for _____ is now part of routine newborn screening in the United States.

20. Transmission of HIV is possible during all stages of infection, even before it can be detected by _____.

21. The use of _____ significantly decreases the risk of HIV transmission to an HIV-seronegative sexual partner.

ANATOMIC STRUCTURES

Identify the following structures of the immune system.

1. Immune system

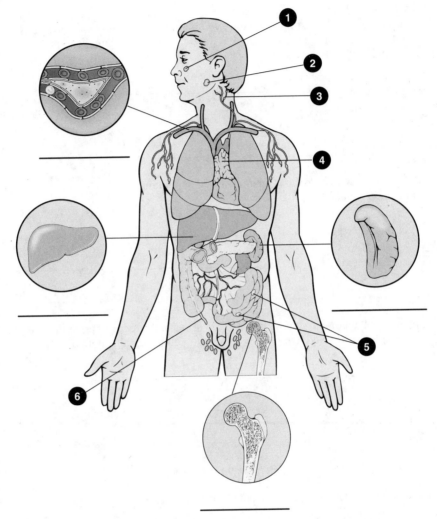

(1) _____   (4) _____

(2) _____   (5) _____

(3) _____   (6) _____

PATIENT SCREENING

For each of the following scenarios, explain how and why you would schedule an appointment or suggest a referral based on the patient's reported symptoms. First review the "Guidelines for Patient-Screening Exercises" found on p. iv in the Introduction

1. A woman calls to discuss a condition her husband is experiencing. She reports that he is complaining of feeling fatigued and experiencing weakness. In addition, she tells you that he has started experiencing chills, has a fever, and is complaining of shortness of breath. She also states that his skin is pale and jaundiced and that he appears to bruise easily. How do you respond to this phone call?

_____

_____

_____

2. A patient previously diagnosed with pernicious anemia calls complaining of an increased weakness and a rapid heart rate. How do you handle this phone call?

_____

_____

_____

3. A patient calls complaining of spitting up blood, blood in his urine, and a reduced amount of urine. He also mentions a recent weight loss, being fatigued, and having a fever. How do you handle this phone call?

_____

_____

_____

4. A female patient calls stating that she is experiencing an unexplained weight loss, fatigue, a persistent low-grade fever, and general malaise. She also mentions joint stiffness, especially on wakening and during periods of inactivity. She requests an appointment for an evaluation and treatment of her symptoms. How do you respond to her?

_____

_____

_____

5. A patient has previously been diagnosed with polymyositis. This patient calls the office complaining of a sudden significant loss of strength and some problems swallowing. How do you handle this phone call?

_____

_____

_____

PATIENT TEACHING

For each scenario below, outline the appropriate patient teaching you would perform. First review the "Guidelines for Patient-Teaching Exercises" found on p. XX in the Introduction.

1. COMMON VARIABLE IMMUNODEFICIENCY (ACQUIRED) HYPOGAMMAGLOBULINEMIA

    Diagnosis of common variable immunodeficiency (acquired) hypogammaglobulinemia has just been confirmed. The physician has printed information for patients about this disorder. How do you handle this patient-teaching opportunity?

    _____

    _____

    _____

2. CHRONIC MUCOCUTANEOUS CANDIDIASIS

    A diagnosis of chronic mucocutaneous candidiasis has just been confirmed. The physician has printed material concerning this disorder. You have been instructed to provide this information to the patient and discuss comfort measures for mouth care. How do you handle this patient-teaching opportunity?

    _____

    _____

    _____

3. IDIOPATHIC THROMBOCYTOPENIC PURPURA

    A child has been diagnosed with idiopathic thrombocytopenic purpura, and infusion therapy is probably going to be prescribed. The physician has printed information regarding this therapy and treatment of this disorder. You are instructed to use this printed information and discuss it with the family. How do you handle this patient-teaching opportunity?

    _____

    _____

    _____

4. RHEUMATOID ARTHRITIS

    A patient with rheumatoid arthritis has just concluded a visit with the physician. The physician has printed material concerning the cause and treatment options for this disorder. You have been instructed to discuss this material with the patient. How do you handle this patient-teaching opportunity?

    _____

    _____

    _____

5. MULTIPLE SCLEROSIS

A patient with multiple sclerosis has experienced an exacerbation of the condition. The physician has printed materials regarding possible treatments of and medications prescribed for this disorder. You are instructed to review this material with the patient. How do you handle this patient-teaching opportunity?

_____

_____

_____

PHARMACOLOGY QUESTIONS

Circle the letter of the choice that best completes the statement or answers the question.

1. Which vitamin is used to treat pernicious anemia?

   a. K

   b. C

   c. E

   d. B_{12}

2. Which medications are not effective for the treatment of systemic lupus erythematosus?

   a. Antiinflammatory

   b. Anticoagulants

   c. Corticosteroids

   d. Immunosuppressants

3. The drug(s) of choice for myasthenia gravis is(are):

   a. Immunosuppressants.

   b. Corticosteroids.

   c. Pyridostigmine (Mestinon).

   d. None of the above.

4. The primary objective of the treatment of rheumatoid arthritis is the reduction of pain and inflammation. Which classification of drug is considered first-line therapy?

   a. Antidepressant

   b. Antiinflammatory

   c. Hormone replacement therapy

   d. Biologic response modifiers

ESSAY QUESTION

Write a response to the following question or statement. Use a separate sheet of paper if more space is needed.

1. Discuss the guidelines that are included in infection control and Universal Precautions and their importance in the safety of the health care worker.

_____

_____

_____

_____

_____

_____

_____

_____

_____

_____

_____

_____

2. Describe the treatment and prognosis of a patient with selective immunoglobulin a deficiency.

_____

_____

_____

_____

_____

_____

_____

_____

_____

_____

_____

_____

_____

3. Discuss the treatment for multiple sclerosis (MS).

_____

_____

_____

_____

_____

_____

_____

_____

_____

_____

_____

4. How did the immune system concept arise?

_____

_____

_____

_____

_____

_____

_____

_____

_____

_____

_____

_____

_____

5. Discuss the three clinically distinct forms of transplant rejection. When does rejection occur and what interventions can be taken?

_____

_____

_____

_____

_____

_____

_____

_____

_____

_____

_____

_____

_____

Circle the letter of the choice that best completes the statement or answers the question.

1. Idiopathic thrombocytopenic anemia involves a deficiency of platelets and:

    a. A decrease in red blood cell count.

    b. A decrease in white blood cell count.

    c. The inability of blood to clot.

    d. None of the above.

2. Active immunity is acquired when a person:

    a. Has a disease.

    b. Receives an immunization.

    c. Is born.

    d. None of the above.

3. Autoimmune diseases occur when:

    a. A person's immune system reacts appropriately to an antigen and homeostasis is maintained.

    b. Antibodies develop and begin to destroy the body's own cells.

    c. A person fails to receive childhood immunizations.

    d. All of the above.

4. Symptoms of butterfly rash, fever, joint pain, malaise, and weight loss are present with:

    a. Scleroderma.

    b. Systemic lupus erythematosus.

    c. Rheumatoid arthritis.

    d. None of the above.

5. Symptoms of inflammation and edema are present at the onset of:

    a. Scleroderma.

    b. Systemic lupus erythematosus.

    c. Rheumatoid arthritis.

    d. None of the above.

6. Symptoms of hardening and shrinking of the skin are associated with:

    a. Scleroderma.

    b. Systemic lupus erythematosus.

    c. Rheumatoid arthritis.

    d. None of the above.

7. Myasthenia gravis is treated with:

    a. Mestinon.

    b. Vitamin B$_{12}$.

    c. Both a and b.

    d. None of the above.

8. The thymus glands produce:

    a. A-cell lymphocytes.

    b. C-cell lymphocytes.

    c. T-cell lymphocytes.

    d. All of the above.

9. HIV is transmitted by:

    a. Sexual contact.

    b. Blood and body fluids.

    c. Both a and b.

    d. None of the above.

10. Selective immunoglobulin A deficiency disease is:

    a. The most common form of immunodeficiency in the general population.

    b. The least common form of immunodeficiency in the general population.

    c. Transmitted by close casual contact.

    d. None of the above.

11. Pernicious anemia is treated with:

    a. Blood transfusions.

    b. Vitamin B$_{12}$.

    c. Plasma.

    d. None of the above.

12. Ankylosing spondylitis primarily affects:

    a. The shoulder.

    b. The spine.

    c. The knee.

    d. All of the above.

13. Multiple sclerosis is an inflammatory disease that attacks:

    a. The joints.

    b. The spinal nerves.

    c. The myelin sheath.

    d. None of the above.

14. Myasthenia gravis is a chronic progressive disease that is characterized by:

    a. Muscle stiffness.

    b. Extreme muscular weakness and progressive fatigue.

    c. Pain.

    d. None of the above.

15. Congenital X-linked agammaglobulinemia:

    a. Is a condition of severe B-cell deficiency.

    b. Affects only males.

    c. Is treated with intravenous infusions of immunoglobulin.

    d. All of the above.

16. Of significant importance in the treatment and prognosis for patients with rheumatoid arthritis is:

    a. Regular vitamin B_{12} injections.

    b. Early aggressive treatment to help prevent deformity.

    c. Blood transfusions.

    d. Vitamin K administration.

17. The patient with Goodpasture's syndrome has:

    a. An autoimmune disease that can cause acute renal failure.

    b. A condition also known as lupus.

    c. Hardening and shrinking of the skin.

    d. Inflammation in various glands of the body.

18. The patient with Sjögren's syndrome has:

    a. An autoimmune disease that can cause acute renal failure.

    b. A condition also known as lupus.

    c. Hardening and shrinking of the skin.

    d. Inflammation in various glands of the body.

19. Although no cure or effective vaccine exists for AIDS, highly active antiretroviral therapy:

    a. Makes transmission of HIV impossible.

    b. Is used in diagnosis of AIDS.

    c. Causes destruction of T cells.

    d. Has significantly prolonged the life span of those infected with AIDS.

20. Currently HIV infection is most often associated with:

    a. Handshaking and hugging.

    b. Homosexual activity.

    c. Heterosexual transmission.

    d. All of the above.

21. The only curative treatment for most types of severe combined immunodeficiency is:

    a. Administration of live vaccines.

    b. Vitamin D.

    c. Antibiotic administration.

    d. Bone marrow transplantation.

22. Transmission of HIV is possible:

    a. Before it can be detected by laboratory tests.

    b. Only when it can be detected by laboratory tests.

    c. During the "window period."

    d. Both a and c.

23. Patients with positive testing results for HIV:

    a. Are encouraged to inform their partner(s) that they may be at high risk for contracting the disease.

    b. Need not inform their sexual partner(s) for 6 months.

    c. Should wash their hands regularly to avoid transmission of the disease.

    d. None of the above.

24. Which autoimmune disease occurs in males only?

    a. DiGeorge's anomaly

    b. X-linked agammaglobulinemia

    c. Wiskott-Aldrich syndrome

    d. Both b and c

25. Testing for which immunodeficiency disease is now part of newborn screening in the United States?

    a. SCID

    b. Polymyositis

    c. CVID

    d. None of the above

26. Graves disease, Hashimoto disease, and Type 1 diabetes involve which system?

    a. Circulatory

    b. Exocrine

    c. Nervous

    d. Endocrine

27. Systemic lupus erythematosus, progressive sclerodema, and Sjogren syndrome involve which system?

    a. Exocrine

    b. Nervous

    c. Immune

    d. Excretory

28. Which symptoms and signs are associated with DiGeorge (thymic hypoplasia or aplasia)?

    a. Abnormally wide, downward-slanting eyes

    b. Severe, recurrent infections with bacteria, viruses, fungi, and protozoa

    c. The thymus and parathyroid glands are absent or underdeveloped

    d. A small mouth

Scenario

Scenario will require students to use critical thinking skills to determine the various possible answers. Some research may be necessary to include an evidence-based answer.

1. There is an order to draw blood on a patient that may or may not have a contagious disease. You apply all universal standard precautions including mask, face shield, gown, gloves. The patient comments, *"Don't you think this is a little extreme, without knowing if I even have any diseases? You make me feel uncomfortable and like I should be isolated from everyone!"*

    A. Explain in detail how to comfort the patient and the reasons for the personal protective equipment.

    _____

    _____

    _____

    _____

    _____

4 Diseases and Conditions of the Endocrine System

WORD DEFINITIONS

Define the following basic medical terms.

1. Anterior _____

2. Assay _____

3. Atrophy _____

4. Copious _____

5. Dysfunction _____

6. Encephalopathy _____

7. Fatigue _____

8. Flatus _____

9. Hyperplasia _____

10. Hyposecretion _____

11. Hypotension _____

12. Inspection _____

13. Palpation _____

14. Palpitation _____

15. Polydipsia _____

16. Polyphagia _____

17. Polyuria _____

18. Specific gravity _____

19. Tremor _____

20. Turgor _____

GLOSSARY TERMS

Define the following chapter glossary terms.

1. Adenoma _____

2. Aerodigestive _____

3. Corticotropin _____

4. Dysphagia _____

5. Endemic _____

6. Epiphyseal _____

7. Goitrogenic _____

8. Hyperglycemia _____

9. Hyperlipidemia _____

10. Hyperparathyroidism _____

11. Hypertrophy _____

12. Idiopathic _____

13. Infarct _____

14. Metastasize _____

15. Panhypopituitarism _____

16. Pathogenesis _____

17. Pruritus _____

18. Radioimmunoassay _____

19. Stridor _____

20. Sulfonylureas _____

21. Syncope _____

SHORT ANSWER

Answer the following questions.

1. Name the master gland of the endocrine system.

   _____

2. Identify the hormones responsible for stimulating secretion of other hormones.

   _____

3. Endocrine diseases result from an abnormal secretion of what?

   _____

4. Name three types of laboratory tests that may be used to evaluate hormone levels.

   _____

5. Acromegaly and gigantism are conditions resulting from an overproduction of which hormone?

_____

6. Identify the term used for the abnormal underdevelopment of the body occurring in children.

_____

7. Is diabetes insipidus more common in males or females?

_____

8. Name the most common endocrine gland to produce a disease, condition, or problem.

_____

9. Identify the hormone released from the pituitary gland that controls the activity of the thyroid gland.

_____

10. Is Hashimoto's disease more common in male or female patients? Cite statistics of incidence in comparing the sexes.

_____

11. Describe the most outstanding clinical feature of Hashimoto's disease.

_____

12. Name the branch of medicine that deals with endocrine disorders.

_____

13. List two examples of ways to ensure ingestion of iodine.

_____

14. Describe the goal of treatment for a patient with Graves' disease.

_____

15. Cite the age range during which cretinism develops.

_____

16. Name the therapeutic agent that is administered to treat myxedema.

_____

17. List the four main types of thyroid cancer.

_____

18. Of the four types, identify the most common type(s) of thyroid cancer.

_____

19. Describe the symptoms of Cushing's syndrome.

_____

_____

20. Explain the treatment for Addison's disease.

_____

_____

_____

21. List five oral medications that are commonly used to treat type 2 diabetes.

_____

22. Name the organs that can be damaged if blood glucose levels are not controlled.

_____

23. Identify the type of diabetes that has its onset during pregnancy.

_____

24. Name the condition associated with documented low blood glucose level and correlating symptoms that resolve with the administration of glucose.

_____

25. At what age is puberty considered precocious in male adolescents?

_____

26. At what age is puberty considered precocious in female adolescents?

_____

27. Identify the hormone responsible for promoting bone and tissue growth.

_____

28. Identify the hormone responsible for regulating skin pigmentation.

_____

29. Name the hormone that causes uterine contractions.

_____

30. Name the hormone that causes development of female secondary sex characteristics.

_____

31. Identify the treatment for when a larger goiter is unresponsive.

_____

FILL IN THE BLANKS

Fill in the blanks with the correct terms. A word list has been provided.

Word List

acute reactive, anaplastic, anterior pituitary adenoma, bone, 2, breakdown, congenital, damage, dilute urine, emergency, excessive calcium, excitability, extreme thirst, eyes, follicle-stimulating hormone, 40, genetic factor, forehead, glands, goiter, gonadal, growth, growth and development, hematocrit, hypothalamus, idiopathic, immune, insomnia, lymphocyte, mental, myxedema, nose, palpitations, pituitary, potassium, puffy, rapid heartbeat, secondary sex, somatotropin (hGH), thick, thymus, thyroxine (T_4), triiodothyronine (T_3), urinary output

1. The action of most hormones is directed at target _____ or at distant receptor sites, thereby regulating critical body functions, such as _____, cellular metabolic rate, _____, and _____.

2. A frequent cause of an oversecretion of human growth hormone is a(an) _____.

3. The cause of hypopituitarism may be a(an) _____ tumor or a tumor of the _____. Some causes are _____ deficiencies and some are acquired, such as _____ to the pituitary gland.

4. The treatment for dwarfism is the administration of _____ until the child reaches the height of 5 feet.

5. Two symptoms of diabetes insipidus are _____ and secretion of _____.

6. A _____ is often the first sign of thyroid disease.

7. The two hormones produced by the thyroid gland are _____ and _____.

8. The cause of Hashimoto's disease is unknown, but a _____ is suggested.

9. A patient with Graves' disease exhibits symptoms of _____, _____, nervousness, _____, and _____. Other symptoms may also be present.

10. A child with cretinism may have symptoms that include _____ and _____ retardation.

11. The face of the patient with _____ becomes bloated, the tongue _____, and the eyelids _____.

12. Thyroid tumors that are undifferentiated, rare, and occur mainly in patients over 60 years of age are _____.

13. Hyperparathyroidism increases the _____ of _____, with the subsequent release of _____ and extracellular fluid.

14. The patient with Addison's disease would exhibit elevated serum _____, blood urea nitrogen, _____ and eosinophil levels, and elevated _____.

15. Patients with type _____ diabetes do not usually require insulin to control blood glucose levels.

16. Approximately 30% to _____% of women who have had gestational diabetes mellitus develop type 2 diabetes within 5 to 10 years after giving birth.

17. An individual with severe symptoms of _____ hypoglycemia requires _____ medical attention.

61

18. Precocious puberty in the male adolescent is exhibited by early development of _____ characteristics, _____ development, and spermatogenesis.

19. In most cases the cause of precocious puberty in females is _____ without associated abnormalities.

20. The hormone responsible for initiating growth of eggs in the ovaries and stimulating spermatogenesis in the testes is called _____.

21. _____ gland that secretes thymosin and promotes development of _____ cells (gland atrophies during adulthood.

22. Some physical characteristics of cretinism include a short _____, broad _____, and small wide-set _____ with puffy eyelids, and a wide-open mouth.

ANATOMIC STRUCTURES

Identify the following structures of the endocrine system.

1. Major glands of the normal endocrine system

(1) _____

(2) _____

(3) _____

(4) _____

(5) _____

(6) _____

(7) _____

(8) _____

(9) _____

(10) _____

11. Which of the following defines the orderly function of the endocrine system?

    a. Thyroid diseases present as functional disturbances that produce excessive or reduced secretions of thyroid hormones—thyroxine (T_4) and triiodothyronine (T_3)—and mass lesions of the thyroid.

    b. Body activities, homeostasis, and the response to stress are communicated and controlled by two distinct but interacting systems: the nervous system and the endocrine system.

    c. The goal of medical management is to achieve normal thyroid function with the lowest possible dose.

    d. Early manifestations include weight gain, hypertension, and emotional instability.

PATIENT SCREENING

For each of the following scenarios, explain how and why you would schedule an appointment or suggest a referral based on the patient's reported symptoms. First review the "Guidelines for Patient-Screening Exercises" found on p. iv in the Introduction.

1. A male patient calls for an appointment. He reports experiencing the sudden onset of excessive thirst and urination. He says that he is thirsty all the time and cannot seem to get enough to drink. How do you respond to this phone call?

_____

_____

_____

2. A female patient calls the office and says she thinks that she has swelling in her neck and is beginning to experience difficulty swallowing. How do you respond to this phone call?

_____

_____

_____

3. An individual calls the office stating that he is experiencing periods of rapid heartbeat and palpitations, insomnia, nervousness, and excitability. He states that, despite excessive appetite and food ingestion, he is losing weight. How do you respond to this call?

_____

_____

_____

4. A woman calls the office stating that her husband, who has been diagnosed with diabetes, is experiencing excessive thirst, nausea, drowsiness, and abdominal pain. She just noticed a fruity odor on his breath. She wants to know what to do. How do you respond to this call?

_____

_____

_____

5. A patient calls the office saying that she has started experiencing weight loss, excessive thirst, excessive hunger, and frequent urination. She also tells you her mother and aunt have diabetes. She says that she just doesn't feel right. How do you respond to this call?

_____

_____

_____

6. A patient call with questions on how hypopituitarism is diagnosed. What information is shared?

_____

_____

_____

_____

_____

_____

PATIENT TEACHING

For each scenario that follows, outline the appropriate patient teaching you would perform. First review the "Guidelines for Patient-Teaching Exercises" found on p. iv in the Introduction.

1. ACROMEGALY
   A diagnosis of acromegaly has been confirmed. The physician (an endocrinologist) has printed materials concerning the disorder. You have been instructed to review the material with the patient and his or her family. How do you handle this patient-teaching opportunity?

_____

_____

_____

2. DIABETES INSIPIDUS

A diagnosis of diabetes insipidus has been confirmed. You are instructed to use available printed material to discuss treatment guidelines with the patient. How do you handle this patient-teaching opportunity?

_____

_____

_____

3. GRAVES' DISEASE

An individual with Graves' disease has been noncompliant with prescribed medications and has experienced an exacerbation of the condition. The physician has decided that the patient requires additional information about the disorder. You are instructed to review the printed materials and guidelines with the patient. How do you handle this patient-teaching opportunity?

_____

_____

_____

4. HYPOTHYROIDISM

A diagnosis of hypothyroidism has just been confirmed. The physician has prescribed a thyroid replacement drug with instructions to take the medication as directed and to schedule a checkup in 6 weeks. In addition, the patient has been told to contact the physician if he or she experiences a rapid heartbeat. How do you handle this patient-teaching opportunity?

_____

_____

_____

5. DIABETES MELLITUS

A previously diagnosed individual with diabetes mellitus has been having difficulty maintaining therapeutic glucose levels. You are instructed to provide instructional material concerning the importance of monitoring glucose levels and possible complications of the disorder. How would you handle this patient-teaching opportunity?

_____

_____

_____

PHARMACOLOGY QUESTIONS

Circle the letter of the choice that best completes the statement or answers the question.

1. Hypothyroidism is usually treated with thyroid replacement hormones. Which of the following is not a type of thyroid replacement?

    a. Levothyroxine (Synthroid)

    b. Thyroid desiccated

    c. Estradiol (Estrace)

    d. None of the above

65

2. Type 2 diabetes can be treated with all of the following therapies except:

   a. Diet and exercise.

   b. Corticosteroids.

   c. Sulfonylurea drugs.

   d. Insulin.

3. Type 1 diabetes can be treated with all of the following therapies except:

   a. Short-acting insulin.

   b. Long-acting insulin.

   c. Insulin pump therapy.

   d. None of the above.

4. If a patient tests his blood glucose level and it is very high (over 300), what would be the fastest way to reduce his blood glucose level?

   a. Insulin

   b. A simple sugar

   c. Metformin (Glucophage)

   d. Acarbase (Precose)

5. Medical treatment of Graves' disease includes:

   a. Antithyroid drugs.

   b. Drugs to block the synthesis of thyroid hormones.

   c. Beta blockers to treat tachycardia.

   d. All of the above.

ESSAY QUESTION

Write a response to the following question or statement. Use a separate sheet of paper if more space is needed.

1. Explain the symptoms and treatment for hypoglycemia. Why is this condition considered serious?

_____

_____

_____

_____

_____

_____

_____

_____

66

_____

_____

_____

_____

_____

_____

2. What are the sign and symptoms of lactic acidosis?

_____

_____

_____

_____

_____

_____

_____

_____

CERTIFICATION EXAMINATION REVIEW

Circle the letter of the choice that best completes the statement or answers the question.

1. Acromegaly is caused by a hypersecretion of human growth hormone that occurs:

   a. After puberty.

   b. Before puberty.

   c. At birth.

   d. None of the above.

2. Inadequate amounts of dietary iodine may be the cause of:

   a. Graves' disease.

   b. A simple nontoxic goiter.

   c. Addison's disease.

   d. None of the above.

3. A calculated diet and exercise, blood and urine testing, and insulin administration are treatments for:

   a. Gestational diabetes.

   b. Diabetes insipidus.

   c. Diabetes mellitus.

   d. None of the above.

4. Hyperglycemia, thirst, nausea, vomiting, and dry skin are all symptoms of:

   a. Diabetic coma.

   b. Insulin shock.

   c. Gestational diabetes.

   d. None of the above.

5. Any dysfunction of the endocrine system may result in a(an):

   a. Increase in secretion of hormones.

   b. Decrease in secretion of hormones.

   c. Both of the above.

   d. None of the above.

6. A conscious person experiencing insulin shock requires:

   a. Insulin.

   b. Glucose.

   c. Simple sugar.

   d. None of the above.

7. Severe hypothyroidism or myxedema has its onset during:

   a. Infancy.

   b. Older childhood.

   c. Adulthood.

   d. Both b and c.

8. Dwarfism is the abnormal underdevelopment of the body or hypopituitarism that occurs in:

   a. Infancy.

   b. Older childhood.

   c. Adulthood.

   d. None of the above.

9. Gigantism is caused from a hypersecretion of human growth hormone that occurs:

   a. Before puberty.

   b. After puberty.

   c. At any age.

   d. At birth.

10. Cushing's syndrome causes symptoms of:

    a. Weight loss, rash, and alopecia.

    b. Fatigue, muscle weakness, and changes in body appearance.

    c. A bright red rash and itching.

    d. None of the above.

68

11. Palpation of a hard, painless lump or nodule on the thyroid gland, vocal cord paralysis, obstructive symptoms, and cervical-lymph adenopathy all indicate:

   a. An evaluation for cancer of the thyroid gland.

   b. A diagnosis of Cushing's syndrome.

   c. A diagnosis of acromegaly.

   d. None of the above.

12. Addison's disease has a gradual onset and involves the:

   a. Parathyroid glands.

   b. Pancreas.

   c. Adrenal glands.

   d. Thyroid gland.

13. Which of the following statements is true regarding myxedema coma?

   a. This condition is a result of severe hyperthyroidism.

   b. This condition is a common one.

   c. Myxedema coma is a medical emergency because it has a high mortality rate.

   d. The patient develops myxedema coma as a result of hypogonadism.

14. Which endocrine gland secretes growth hormone (GH)?

   a. The anterior pituitary

   b. The thymus gland

   c. The thyroid gland

   d. The pineal gland

15. The gland that regulates the metabolism of calcium is:

   a. The posterior pituitary.

   b. The pancreas.

   c. The parathyroid gland.

   d. The pineal gland.

16. A congenital hypothyroid condition in which the thyroid gland is absent or thyroid hormone is not synthesized by the thyroid gland; this causes mental and growth retardation in the infant or young child. This condition is known as:

   a. Cretinism.

   b. Hypothyroidism.

   c. Myxedema.

   d. Acromegaly.

17. Which of the following defines the orderly function of the endocrine system?

    a. Thyroid diseases present as functional disturbances that produce excessive or reduced secretions of thyroid hormones—thyroxine (T_4) and triiodothyronine (T_3)—and mass lesions of the thyroid.

    b. Body activities, homeostasis, and the response to stress are communicated and controlled by two distinct but interacting systems: the nervous system and the endocrine system.

    c. The goal of medical management is to achieve normal thyroid function with the lowest possible dose.

    d. Early manifestations include weight gain, hypertension, and emotional instability

18. In the endocrine system, which gland produces quick-acting "fight or flight" responses during stress; increases blood pressure, heart rate, and blood glucose level; and dilates bronchioles?

    a. Pancreas

    b. Adrenal medulla

    c. Thyroid

    d. Parathyroid

19. Acromegaly is usually seem in people at which age?

    a. Children under 5 years old.

    b. It is often seen in people 30 to 40 years old.

    c. In adolescence between 12 and 18 years old.

    d. Over the age of 60.

Scenario

Scenario will require students to use critical thinking skills to determine the various possible answers. Some research may be necessary to include an evidence-based answer.

The office staff will be taking part in a free local health fair and have been asked to educate the community. The office sets up a booth to help the community in groups of 10 at a time.

1. The first group of 10 visitors are parents that need information regarding recognizing symptoms associated with, and caring for kids and teens who have, type 2 diabetes. How will this be managed?

2. The second group of 10 visitors are the kids and teens that need information on how to help prevent type 2 diabetes. How will this be managed?

5 Diseases and Disorders of the Eye and Ear

Define the following basic medical terms.

1. Arteritis _____

2. Bilateral _____

3. Dilated _____

4. Edema _____

5. Excision _____

6. Hemorrhage _____

7. Hyperopia _____

8. Hypertrophied _____

9. Intracranial _____

10. Intraocular _____

11. Meningitis _____

12. Myopia _____

13. Postoperative _____

14. Proliferative _____

15. Strabismus _____

16. Systemic _____

17. Topical _____

18. Vertigo _____

19. Blepharitis _____

20. Cryotherapy _____

21. Labyrinth _____

22. Myringotomy _____

23. Otoscopy _____

24. Retinopathy _____

GLOSSARY TERMS

Define the following chapter glossary terms.

1. Amblyopia _____

2. Analgesics _____

3. Ankylosis _____

4. Audiogram _____

5. Diplopia _____

6. Histoplasmosis _____

7. Laser photocoagulation _____

8. Macula _____

9. Photophobia _____

10. Purulent _____

11. Seborrhea _____

12. Tinnitus _____

13. Tonometry _____

14. Toxoplasmosis _____

15. Tympanic membrane _____

SHORT ANSWER

Answer the following questions.

1. Identify the concentric layers of the eyeball that are its primary structure.

_____

2. Name the colorless transparent structure located on the front of the eye.

_____

3. List the way that hearing loss is classified.

_____

4. Explain the symptoms associated with otosclerosis.

_____

5. Name the canal that leads from the middle ear to the nasopharynx.

_____

6. Identify the structure in the ear that is responsible for helping a person maintain balance.

_____

7. Cite the shape of the normal eyeball.

_____

8. Name the sensory receptive cells in the retina that make the detection of color and fine detail possible.

_____

9. Identify the wax-like secretion that is produced by the glands of the external ear canal.

_____

10. Name the jellylike fluid found in the cavity behind the lens of the eye.

_____

11. Name the internal elastic structure of the eye that focuses images both near and far.

_____

12. What is the cause of a cholesteatoma?

_____

13. If the eyeball is abnormally short, name the condition that occurs.

_____

14. If the eyeball is abnormally long, name the condition that occurs.

_____

15. Identify the cause of astigmatism.

_____

16. List the primary symptoms of refractive errors.

_____

17. Name the most common type of nystagmus.

_____

18. Identify the bacteria that are the common cause of styes.

_____

19. List the symptoms of keratitis.

_____

20. Explain the most common cause of cataracts.

_____

21. Is there a cure for macular degeneration?

_____

22. Identify the disorder of the retinal blood vessels that may develop in a person who has diabetes.

_____

23. Explain the steps that may be used to remove impacted cerumen.

_____

_____

24. List the four most common causes of a ruptured eardrum.

_____

_____

25. Name the three eye diseases that are leading causes of blindness.

_____

26. List causes of infective otitis media.

_____

27. List symptoms of otitis media.

_____

28. List common treatment options for otitis media.

_____

29. List common symptoms of Meniere's disease.

_____

30. Identify the main symptom of labyrinthitis.

_____

31. List possible causes of ruptured tympanic membrane.

_____

74

FILL IN THE BLANKS

Fill in the blanks with the correct terms. A word list has been provided. Words used twice are indicated with a (2).

Word List

age, astigmatism, bacterial, blood glucose, cerumen, chemicals, choroid, cornea, distant, esotropia, eye, familiar, hearing loss, herpes simplex, hyperopia, light, media, metastasize, myopia, pain (2), position, presbyopia, pressure, routine ophthalmic, redness, retina, smoke, strabismus, surface, swelling, tinnitus, viral, vision, vitreous humor, vomiting, weakness, white

1. The iris or colored portion of the eye helps regulate the amount of _____ that enters the eye.

2. The large cavity behind the lens of the eye contains a jellylike fluid called the _____.

3. Four main refractive errors that result when the eye is unable to focus light effectively on the retina are

   _____, _____, _____, and _____.

4. The patient with myopia can see objects that are near but experiences difficulty seeing objects that are

   _____.

5. _____ is the failure of the eyes to look in the same direction at the same time, which primarily occurs

   because of _____ in the nerves stimulating the muscles that control the _____ of the eye.

6. In _____ both eyes turn inward; in exotropia both eyes turn outward.

7. The symptoms of a stye are _____, _____, _____, and formation of pus at the site.

8. Keratitis is frequently caused by an infection resulting from the _____ _____ virus.

9. Allergies or exposure to _____, dust, or _____ can cause nonulcerative blepharitis.

10. Blepharoptosis occurs at any _____; is often _____; and, if severe, blocks the

    _____ of the affected eye.

11. Infection, either _____ or _____, can cause conjunctivitis.

12. A corneal abrasion is the painful loss of _____ epithelium or the outer layer of the _____.

13. A cataract may become visible, giving the pupil a _____, opaque appearance.

14. The best way to detect glaucoma is to have periodic _____ examinations.

15. Common symptoms of ear diseases and conditions that should receive medical attention include _____,

    ear _____ or _____, _____, vertigo, nausea, and _____.

16. Impacted _____ may harden and block sound waves, resulting in decreased hearing.

17. Otitis _____ is the most frequent reason for visits to the physician by children.

18. Diabetic retinopathy occurs in those with diabetes who do not control their _____ levels.

75

19. Retinal detachment is a separation of the _____ from the _____.

20. Many types of cancer are known to _____ to the _____.

ANATOMIC STRUCTURES

Identify the structures in the following anatomic diagrams.

1. Normal eye

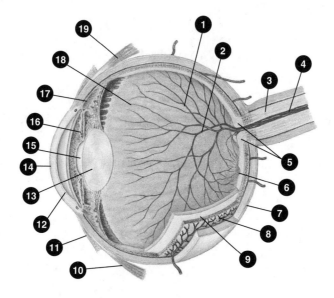

(1) _____

(2) _____

(3) _____

(4) _____

(5) _____

(6) _____

(7) _____

(8) _____

(9) _____

(10) _____

(11) _____

(12) _____

(13) _____

(14) _____

(15) _____

(16) _____

(17) _____

(18) _____

(19) _____

2. The visual pathway

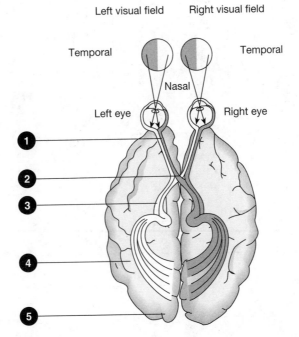

(1) _____

(2) _____

(3) _____

(4) _____

(5) _____

Chapter **5** **Diseases and Disorders of the Eye and Ear**

3. Normal ear

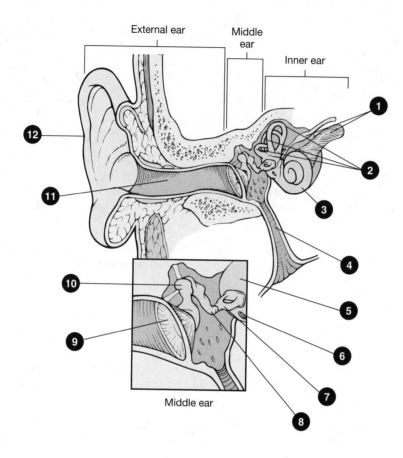

(1) _____

(2) _____

(3) _____

(4) _____

(5) _____

(6) _____

(7) _____

(8) _____

(9) _____

(10) _____

(11) _____

(12) _____

4. Labyrinth or inner ear

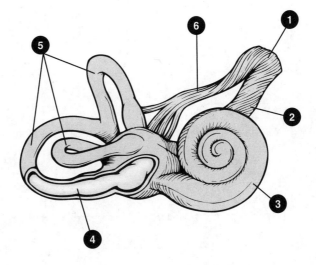

(1) _____

(2) _____

(3) _____

(4) _____

(5) _____

(6) _____

PATIENT SCREENING

For each of the following scenarios, explain how and why you would schedule an appointment or suggest a referral based on the patient's reported symptoms. First review the "Guidelines for Patient-Screening Exercises" found on p. iv in the Introduction.

1. A patient calls in describing a sensation of constantly having something in her right eye. She also states that pain and tearing prevent her from wearing her contact lens in that eye. How do you handle this call?

_____

_____

_____

2. A patient calls advising that he is experiencing changes in his vision and sensitivity to light. How do you handle this call?

_____

_____

_____

Chapter **5** **Diseases and Disorders of the Eye and Ear**

3. A patient calls reporting that she is experiencing reduced vision, especially loss of sharpness in her central vision. How do you respond to this call?

_____

_____

_____

4. A patient calls the office and tells you that he suddenly is having flashes of light along with floating spots in the left eye. How do you respond to this call?

_____

_____

_____

5. A father calls the office to report that his child is experiencing ear pain, has a fever, and appears to have diminished hearing. How do you handle this call?

_____

_____

_____

6. A wife calls reporting that her husband is experiencing a sudden onset of extreme vertigo and an elevated temperature. She adds that his balance is affected and he is also experiencing nausea and vomiting. How do you respond to this call?

_____

_____

_____

PATIENT TEACHING

For each scenario below, outline the appropriate patient teaching you would perform. First review the "Guidelines for Patient-Teaching Exercises" found on p. iv in the Introduction.

1. STYE

   A patient has just been diagnosed with having a stye on the eyelid. Eye compresses and topical antibiotics have been prescribed. You are instructed to provide the patient with instructions regarding the application of compresses and topical eye medications. How would you handle this patient-teaching opportunity?

_____

_____

_____

_____

_____

2. **KERATITIS**

A diagnosis of keratitis has been made. The physician instructs you to use printed materials to explain proper administration of eye medications and to reinforce the importance of good handwashing before touching an eye. How do you handle this patient-teaching opportunity?

_____

_____

_____

_____

_____

3. **CONJUNCTIVITIS**

A patient with conjunctivitis has been advised to use cool compresses on both eyes for comfort. Topical ophthalmic medications have also been prescribed for therapeutic treatment. You have been instructed to advise the patient on how to apply the cool compresses and medications. How would you handle this patient-teaching opportunity?

_____

_____

_____

_____

_____

4. **GLAUCOMA**

A patient has just been diagnosed with glaucoma. (Type is insignificant in this situation.) You have been instructed to discuss treatment regimen with the patient. How do you handle this patient-teaching opportunity?

_____

_____

_____

_____

_____

5. **IMPACTED CERUMEN**

A child has been experiencing diminished hearing and has been complaining of slight pain in the ears. A diagnosis of impacted cerumen is made. You are instructed to reinforce appropriate cleansing of the ear canal. How do you handle this patient-teaching opportunity?

_____

_____

_____

81

_____

_____

6. SWIMMER'S EAR

Two children in a family have been experiencing swimmer's ear since the family installed a swimming pool. Antibiotic ear drops have been prescribed on the past two occurrences. During a recent visit, a discussion took place concerning the importance of drying the ears thoroughly after swimming. Upon questioning, the children confirmed they were not taking time to completely dry the outer ear canal. How do you handle this patient-teaching opportunity?

_____

_____

_____

_____

_____

PHARMACOLOGY QUESTIONS

Circle the letter of the choice that best completes the statement or answers the question.

1. Treatment of more severe blepharitis may include which of the following?

    a. Oral indomethacin

    b. Antibiotic ophthalmic ointment or drops

    c. Conjugated estrogen (Premarin)

    d. Terbinafine ointment (Bactroban)

2. Bacterial conjunctivitis is best treated with:

    a. Clopidogrel.

    b. Clotrimazole (Lotrimin).

    c. Topical antibiotics or systemically.

    d. Prednisone.

3. Which of the following medications can be used for the treatment of glaucoma?

    a. Betaxolol (Betagan)

    b. Timolol (Timoptic)

    c. Latanoprost (Xalatan)

    d. All of the above

4. To achieve best results in the treatment of open-angle glaucoma, the patient should be instructed to:

    a. Apply cold compresses to the eye twice a day.

    b. Use the prescribed eye medication on a regular basis and not miss doses.

    c. Use the prescribed eye medication only if headache or blurred vision is present.

    d. Follow the prescribed course of topical or, in severe cases, systemic steroids.

5. Patients diagnosed with macular degeneration are commonly prescribed which combination of vitamins?

    a. Vitamins A, C, E, and zinc

    b. Vitamins B1, B6, B12, and iron

    c. Vitamins K

    d. Thiamin, riboflavin, and cyanocobalamin

6. Impacted cerumen is best removed with which of the following medications?

    a. Hydrogen peroxide

    b. Q-tips

    c. Antibiotic-steroid combo

    d. Benzocaine drops

7. Otitis media may be treated with which medication?

    a. Ibuprofen

    b. Pseudoephedrine (Sudafed)

    c. Sulfamethoxazole/trimethoprim

    d. All of the above

8. Meniere's disease can be treated with which of the following medications?

    a. Naproxen sod (Naprosyn)

    b. Phenazopyridine (Pyridium)

    c. Docusate sod (Colace)

    d. Meclizine (Antivert)

9. Drug therapy used in the treatment of mastoiditis includes:

    a. Antibiotic or sulfonamide therapy.

    b. Hydrogen peroxide.

    c. Latanoprost (Xalatan).

    d. Prednisone.

10. Treatment of benign paroxysmal positional vertigo includes:

    a. Antibiotics.

    b. Sulfonamides.

    c. Antihistamines, anticholinergics, and benzodiazepines.

    d. Bed rest for several days.

11. Treatment for labyrinthitis includes:

    a. Bed rest.

    b. Tranquilizers, antiemetics, and/or antibiotics for infection.

    c. Antihistamines and/or corticosteroids.

    d. All of the above.

12. There are several treatments for glaucoma, such as medication, beta-blockers, alpha-adrenergic agents, and different types of laser treatment. What could be a setback when a patient is taking a beta-blocker?

_____

_____

_____

_____

_____

13. Many systemic medications taken for a variety of diseases can have ocular side effects. It is important for patients taking certain systemic medications to be monitored periodically for ocular toxicity. What medications should be monitored and for which disease?

_____

_____

_____

_____

ESSAY QUESTIONS

Write a response to the following question or statement. Use a separate sheet of paper if more space is needed.

1. Discuss the symptoms, causes, and treatment for a ruptured tympanic membrane.

_____

_____

_____

_____

_____

_____

_____

_____

_____

_____

_____

_____

_____

_____

2. Write a description of points to stress in patient teaching for a person diagnosed with macular degeneration.

_____

_____

_____

_____

_____

_____

_____

_____

_____

_____

_____

_____

3. Discuss benign paroxysmal positional vertigo, describing the sensations of vertigo.

_____

_____

_____

_____

_____

_____

_____

_____

_____

_____

_____

_____

_____

_____

4. Discuss causes of sensorineural hearing loss.

_____

_____

_____

_____

_____

_____

_____

_____

_____

_____

_____

_____

_____

5. Identify eight eyelid disorders

(1) _____

(2) _____

(3) _____

(4) _____

(5) _____

(6) _____

(7) _____

(8) _____

6. Name the three intrinsic smooth muscles of the eye.

   _____

   _____

   _____

7. Discuss the symptoms and signs of Episcleritis/Scleritis including the following questions: (a) Is only one eye affected or both? (b) Is it painful? (c) Can it cause blindness?

   _____

   _____

   _____

8. What is the descriptive difference between presbyopia and nystagmus?

   _____

   _____

   _____

   _____

9. Contrast the prognosis of children and an adult with strabismus?

   _____

   _____

   _____

CERTIFICATION EXAMINATION REVIEW

Circle the letter of the choice that best completes the statement or answers the question.

1. When the eye is unable to focus light effectively, which of the following may result?

   a. Hyperopia

   b. Myopia

   c. Presbyopia

   d. All of the above

87

2. Laser surgery, contact lenses, or eyeglasses would be treatment for:

    a. Folliculitis.

    b. Conjunctivitis.

    c. Refractive errors.

    d. All of the above.

3. A stye is an:

    a. Inflammation of the conjunctiva.

    b. Inflammation of the sebaceous glands of the eyelid.

    c. Inflammation of the retina.

    d. Inflammation of the meibomian glands.

4. Conjunctivitis is an:

    a. Inflammation of the conjunctiva, the mucous membrane that covers the anterior portion of the eyeball and also lines the eyelid.

    b. Inflammation of the hair follicle of the eyelid.

    c. Inflammation of the retina.

    d. Inflammation of the cornea.

5. Infection, irritation, allergies, or chemicals may be the cause of:

    a. Hyperopia.

    b. Myopia.

    c. Conjunctivitis.

    d. All of the above.

6. Diabetic retinopathy and glaucoma are major causes of _____ in the United States.

    a. Blindness

    b. Hearing loss

    c. Retinal detachment

    d. Malignancies

7. Otosclerosis is an ankylosing of the:

    a. Labyrinth.

    b. Stapes.

    c. Eyelid.

    d. Tympanic membrane.

8. Labyrinthitis is an inflammation of the:

    a. Stapes.

    b. Conjunctiva.

    c. Semicircular canal.

    d. Tympanic membrane.

9. Otosclerosis, impacted cerumen, and otitis media may be the etiology of:

   a. Conductive hearing loss.

   b. Sensorineural hearing loss.

   c. Both a and b.

   d. Neither a nor b.

10. The internal _____ of the eye is elastic and can focus images both near and far.

    a. Sclera

    b. Iris

    c. Lens

    d. Retina

11. The most common cause of blindness in the United States is:

    a. Uveitis.

    b. Retinal detachment.

    c. Macular degeneration.

    d. Cataract.

12. Treatment for an acute attack of Meniere's disease would include:

    a. Diuretics, antiemetics, anticholinergics, antihistamines, and mild sedatives.

    b. Increased fluid intake.

    c. Limiting the amount of caffeine and alcohol in the diet and stopping smoking.

    d. Both a and c.

13. Strabismus should be treated as soon as possible to:

    a. Prevent hordeolum (stye).

    b. Prevent conjunctivitis.

    c. Prevent amblyopia.

    d. Prevent infection.

14. Treatment of swimmer's ear includes:

    a. Thoroughly cleaning and drying the ear after swimming.

    b. Antihistamines.

    c. Antifungal cream.

    d. Myringotomy.

15. Causes of ruptured tympanic membrane include:

    a. Infection.

    b. Blow to the ear.

    c. Nearby explosion.

    d. All of the above.

16. Which of the extrinsic muscles of the eye rotates the eyeball downward and medially; adducts, and causes the eye to look up?

    a. Lateral rectus and medial rectus.

    b. Inferior rectus and superior rectus.

    c. Inferior oblique and superior oblique.

    d. Lateral rectus and inferior oblique.

17. Which major part of the eye's function is a light receptor that transforms optic signals into nerve impulses, distinguishes light from dark and perceives shape and movement, and color vision?

    a. Cornea

    b. Choroid

    c. Lens

    d. Optic nerve

18. Macular degeneration is a progressive deterioration or breakdown of which f the following?

    a. Choroid

    b. Retinal vein

    c. Retinal artery

    d. Macula

Scenario

Scenario will require students to use critical thinking skills to determine the various possible answers. Some research may be necessary to include an evidence-based answer.

1. Explain eye care to a patient is diagnosed with diabetes mellitus.

    a. Why is it important that they have a comprehensive ophthalmologic examination yearly?

    _____

    _____

    _____

    _____

    _____

    b. How would you convey the importance of an annual exam to the patient?

    _____

    _____

    _____

    _____

    _____

WORD DEFINITIONS

Define the following basic medical terms.

1. Albinism _____

2. Colic _____

3. Edema _____

4. Epidemic _____

5. Erythema _____

6. Excision _____

7. Exudate _____

8. Fissure _____

9. Hyperplastic _____

10. Hypertrophic _____

11. Lesion _____

12. Peripheral _____

13. Psychosis _____

14. Sebaceous _____

15. Spore _____

16. Superficial _____

17. Unilateral _____

18. Wheal _____

19. Cellulitis _____

20. Comedo _____

21. Idopathic _____

22. Papule _____

GLOSSARY TERMS

Define the following chapter glossary terms.

1. Asymptomatic _____

2. Comedones _____

3. Debriding _____

4. Dermatomes _____

5. Erythema _____

6. Exacerbations _____

7. Idiopathic _____

8. Keratin _____

9. Keratolytic _____

10. Melanin _____

11. Papules _____

12. Plaques _____

13. Pustules _____

14. Sebum _____

15. Toxic _____

16. Vesicles _____

SHORT ANSWER

Answer the following questions.

1. List the functions of the skin.

   _____

2. Describe the symptoms of psoriasis.

   _____

3. Identify the oily secretion that is produced by the sebaceous glands.

   _____

4. On what are diagnoses of cutaneous diseases based?

   _____

5. Identify another name for a skin tag.

   _____

6. Which type of skin cancer is the most prevalent form of cancer worldwide?

_____

7. Identify the bacteria that cause impetigo.

_____

8. List examples of dermatophytosis.

_____

9. List examples of common benign skin tumors.

_____

10. Identify the other name for a mole.

_____

11. Are keloids benign or malignant?

_____

12. When do keloids form?

_____

13. At what age will cradle cap resolve if left untreated?

_____

14. Name the test that is used to identify specific irritants or allergens that cause contact dermatitis.

_____

15. List three things that may cause eczema to flare up.

_____

16. Explain the goal of treatment for psoriasis.

_____

17. Identify the other name for herpes zoster.

_____

18. Cite the other name for a furuncle.

_____

19. Which area of the body is usually affected by cellulitis?

_____

Chapter **6** **Diseases and Conditions of the Integumentary System**

20. Describe the appearance of a ringworm lesion.

_____

21. Identify the area of the body affected by tinea unguium.

_____

22. Identify the area of the body affected by tinea pedis.

_____

23. Which sex is more at risk for tinea cruris?

_____

24. Cite the statistics for lesion occurrence of basal cell carcinoma on the face.

_____

25. Cite the statistics for 5-year survival rate of nonmelanoma skin cancer.

_____

26. Name the special cells in the skin that produce melanin.

_____

27. What color eyes would a person with albinism have?

_____

28. What is the prognosis for alopecia that results from the aging process or heredity?

_____

29. State the cause of warts.

_____

30. List some of the likely causes of deformed or discolored nails.

_____

31. List the three main structural layers of the skin.

_____

32. List typical manifestations of forms of dermatitis.

_____

33. List common presenting symptoms of skin conditions.

_____

34. Describe a decubitus ulcer.

_____

35. List the ABCDEs of malignant melanoma.

_____

36. Vitiligo, melisma, hemangiomas, and nevi are forms of what?

_____

37. Localized hyperplastic areas of the stratum corneum layer of the epidermis are called what?

_____

38. List the three ways in which contact dermatitis develops.

_____

FILL IN THE BLANKS

Fill in the blanks with the correct terms. A word list has been provided.

Word List
benign, blood vessels, discontinued, epidermis, greasy papules, growths, hives, hormonal, hydrocortisone, insulation, itching, keratin, keratoses, largest, melanin, middle, minoxidil (Rogaine), pityriasis, pregnancy, purple, red, redness, subcutaneous layer,

1. The skin is one of the _____ organs in size.

2. The dermis is the _____ layer of the skin.

3. The _____ is the outer thin layer of the skin that is responsible for the production of _____ and _____.

4. The third layer of the skin is the _____, a thick, fat-containing section that provides _____ for the body against heat loss.

5. Seborrheic dermatitis can be treated effectively with topical _____ cream.

6. Urticaria, or _____, is associated with symptoms of severe _____, followed by the appearance of _____ and an area of swelling.

7. Albinism is a rare _____ condition.

8. Melasma occurs in some women during _____ changes. The condition disappears after _____ or when oral contraceptive use is _____.

9. Hemangiomas are _____ lesions of proliferating _____ that produce a _____, blue, or _____ color.

10. Seborrheic _____ are benign _____ originating in the epidermis, clinically appearing as tan brown _____ or plaques appearing to be pasted on the skin.

11. A fungal infection that causes patches of flaky light or dark skin to develop on the trunk of the body is called _____.

12. The treatment that is showing promise for male pattern baldness is _____ preparations used topically in cream and spray forms.

95

Identify the structures of the following anatomic diagram.

1. Normal skin

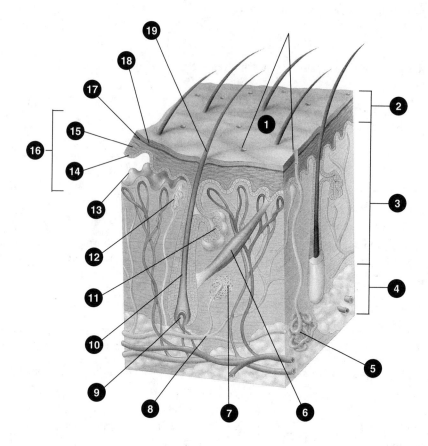

(1) _____   (11) _____

(2) _____   (12) _____

(3) _____   (13) _____

(4) _____   (14) _____

(5) _____   (15) _____

(6) _____   (16) _____

(7) _____   (17) _____

(8) _____   (18) _____

(9) _____   (19) _____

(10) _____

PATIENT SCREENING

For each of the following scenarios, explain how and why you would schedule an appointment or suggest a referral based on the patient's reported symptoms. First review the "Guidelines for Patient-Screening Exercises" found on p. iv in the Introduction.

1. The mother of a 10-year-old child calls in to request an appointment for her daughter who has seeping eruptions on her elbows and knees. She also says that the child is experiencing constant itching. How do you handle this phone call?

   _____

   _____

   _____

2. A patient calls complaining of severe itching of the arms, hands, and trunk accompanied by a red rash. This situation has occurred in the past 2 hours and is getting progressively worse. How do you handle this call?

   _____

   _____

   _____

3. A patient's wife calls in stating that her husband has an onset of excruciating pain on the right side in the middle of the trunk. She says it appears that there are small blisterlike eruptions over the area on the right side of the body and he needs help as soon as possible. How do you handle this call?

   _____

   _____

   _____

4. A mother calls reporting her daughter has just come home from school with areas on her legs and arms that have small blisters surrounded with small blisterlike formations. She says that the child is continuously scratching the areas and they are getting worse. She requests an appointment for the next morning, saying she will keep the child home from school until seen by the physician. When do you schedule the child to be seen?

   _____

   _____

   _____

5. A female patient calls stating that she has a sore on her right shoulder that has refused to heal completely and has occurrences of bleeding. She states that the sore is about an inch in diameter and has irregular edges. She requests an appointment for assessment of the sore. How do you schedule the appointment?

   _____

   _____

   _____

PATIENT TEACHING

For each scenario below, outline the appropriate patient teaching you would perform. First review the "Guidelines for Patient-Teaching Exercises" found on p. iv in the Introduction.

1. CONTACT DERMATITIS

A patient has just been seen for the second time in 3 weeks for contact dermatitis. The area is now showing signs of a developing infection. The physician instructs you to reinforce his instructions about avoiding the trigger substance and trying to avoid scratching the area. How do you handle the patient-teaching opportunity?

_____

_____

_____

2. ACNE

A teenage patient has experienced an exacerbation of acne. Topical and oral medications have been prescribed. You have been instructed to provide the patient with printed information regarding the treatment of acne. How do you handle this patient-teaching opportunity?

_____

_____

_____

3. DERMATOPHYTOSIS

A patient has been diagnosed with athlete's foot. You have been instructed to provide him or her with printed information regarding the treatment of this condition. How do you handle this patient-teaching opportunity?

_____

_____

_____

4. SCABIES AND PEDICULOSIS

A patient was sent home from school with the possibility of head lice. You have been instructed to provide the parents and patient with printed information regarding this condition. How will you handle this patient-teaching opportunity?

_____

_____

_____

5. SKIN CANCER

A patient has been seen for several skin lesions. Some are diagnosed as being benign. One is suspicious in nature, and the patient is referred to a dermatologist for further assessment and treatment. You are instructed to provide the patient with printed information concerning skin lesions and to encourage the use of sunscreen. How do you handle this patient-teaching opportunity?

_____

_____

_____

6. IMPETIGO

Discuss how to manage teaching a patient about the causes of impetigo causes and treatment plan for the disease?

_____

_____

_____

PHARMACOLOGY QUESTIONS

Circle the letter of the choice that best completes the statement or answers the question.

1. Which of the following medications is not used to treat atopic dermatitis (eczema)?

   a. Diazepam (Valium)

   b. Diphenhydramine (Benadryl)

   c. Tacrolimus (Protopic)

   d. Disopyramide (Norpace)

2. Acne vulgaris may be treated with:

   a. Tretinoin (Retin-A).

   b. Antibiotics.

   c. Isotretinoin (Accutane).

   d. All of the above.

3. Antiviral therapy is commonly used to treat shingles. Which of the following is not an antiviral medication?

   a. Acyclovir (Zovirax)

   b. Capsaicin (Zostrix)

   c. Famciclovir (Famvir)

   d. Valacyclovir (Valtrex)

4. If treating a patient with a case of impetigo, which systemic antibiotic would be best?

   a. Penicillin

   b. Metronidazole (Flagyl)

   c. Mupirocin (Bactroban)

   d. Tetracycline

5. Which of the following would not be used for the treatment of cellulitis?

   a. Penicillin

   b. Medroxyprogesterone (Provera)

   c. Codeine

   d. Acetaminophen (Tylenol)

6. Ringworm (tinea corporis) is treated with which of the following?

   a. Permethrin (Elimite)

   b. Mebendazole (Vermox)

   c. Terbinafine (Lamisil)

   d. Pyrantel (Pin X)

7. Head lice can be treated with which of the following?

   a. Lindane shampoo

   b. Fine-tooth comb

   c. Permethrin (Elimite)

   d. All of the above

ESSAY QUESTION

Write a response to the following question or statement. Use a separate sheet of paper if more space is needed.

1. Describe the cause, symptoms, and treatment for herpes zoster (shingles).

_____

_____

_____

_____

_____

_____

_____

_____

_____

_____

_____

_____

_____

2. Describe the cause, symptoms, and treatment of rosacea.

_____

_____

_____

_____

_____

_____

_____

_____

_____

_____

_____

_____

_____

3. What is the descriptive difference between psoriasis and rosacea?

_____

_____

_____

_____

4. If decubitus ulcers are not diagnosed and treated in early stages, what complications may develop?

_____

_____

_____

_____

5. In which individuals would you expect find the greatest incidence of scabies and pediculosis?

_____

_____

_____

_____

6. What often is the cause and body location of acrochordon (Skin Tag)?

_____

_____

_____

_____

7. Which eye problems may accompany albinism?

_____

_____

_____

_____

8. There are several treatments available for abnormal sun tanning, including surgical and nonsurgical skin resurfacing, Injectable fillers, Botulinum toxin (BTX), and Botox (Allergan, Inc.). What are some of the warnings patients should be made aware of in applying these treatments?

_____

_____

_____

_____

9. Explain the symptoms and signs of three most often seen Verrucae (warts).

_____

_____

_____

_____

10. How does the skin function in connection with common skin conditions?

_____

_____

_____

_____

_____

_____

_____

_____

CERTIFICATION EXAMINATION REVIEW

Circle the letter of the choice that best completes the statement or answers the question.

1. *Streptococcus* or *Staphylococcus* is a bacterium that can cause the skin infection called:

    a. Psoriasis.

    b. Eczema.

    c. Impetigo.

    d. Rosacea.

2. Atopic dermatitis is another name for _____, a skin infection that tends to occur in people who have a family history of allergic conditions.

    a. Psoriasis

    b. Eczema

    c. Impetigo

    d. Rosacea

3. Cradle cap is a type of seborrheic dermatitis that is seen in:

    a. Infants.

    b. Teenagers.

    c. Adults.

    d. All of the above.

4. Good skin care, early ambulation, and position changes every 2 hours are all considered preventive measures to reduce the likelihood of developing:

    a. Herpes zoster.

    b. Decubitus ulcers.

    c. Atopic dermatitis.

    d. Epidermal cysts.

103

5. The two most common parasitic infections to infest humans are:

   a. Herpes zoster and impetigo.

   b. Atopic dermatitis and seborrheic dermatitis.

   c. Scabies and pediculosis.

   d. Pityriasis and vitiligo.

6. Malignant melanoma is the most serious type of:

   a. Skin cancer.

   b. Fungal infection.

   c. Parasitic infection.

   d. Dermatophytoses.

7. A furuncle is an abscess that involves the entire hair follicle and:

   a. Underlying muscle tissue.

   b. The epidermis.

   c. The adjacent subcutaneous tissue.

   d. Underlying bone.

8. Manifestations of dermatophytosis include:

   a. Tinea capitis, tinea corporis, tinea pedis, and tinea cruris.

   b. Scabies and pediculosis.

   c. Albinism and vitiligo.

   d. All of the above.

9. The patient with psoriasis exhibits symptoms of:

   a. A fine red rash that itches.

   b. Large furuncles and a fine red rash.

   c. Thick, flaky red patches of various sizes covered with white silvery scales.

   d. Extremely painful vesicles.

10. The transmission of lice and scabies from one person to another is:

    a. Difficult.

    b. Easy with close physical contact.

    c. Only possible if two people live in the same house.

    d. Prevented by using soap and water.

11. Contact dermatitis may be caused by:

    a. Exposure.

    b. Sensitization.

    c. Photoallergy.

    d. All of the above.

12. Urticaria is the result of:

   a. Localized hyperplastic areas of the stratum corneum layer of the epidermis.

   b. An acute hypersensitivity and the release of histamine.

   c. A chronic superficial fungal infection of the skin.

   d. Abnormal skin pigmentation.

13. Hemangiomas are a form of:

   a. Abnormal skin pigmentation.

   b. Alopecia.

   c. Skin cancer.

   d. Acne.

14. Rosacea is a type of:

   a. Chronic inflammatory disorder of the facial skin.

   b. Acute hypersensitivity and the release of histamine.

   c. Chronic superficial fungal infection of the skin.

   d. Skin cancer.

15. Warts, a cutaneous manifestation of the human papillomavirus (HPV) infection, are:

   a. Localized hyperplastic areas of the stratum corneum layer of the epidermis.

   b. An inflammatory reaction of the hair follicles.

   c. Spread by touch or contact with the skin shed from a wart.

   d. Also termed *vitiligo*.

16. Folliculitis is an inflammation of:

   a. Hair follicles.

   b. Sebaceous glands.

   c. Fissure.

   d. Comedo.

17. Dark pigment of skin found in the basal layer of the skin is:

   a. Paronychia.

   b. Melanin.

   c. Sebum.

   d. Melasma.

18. Tinea pedis is also called:

   a. Ringworm.

   b. Jock itch.

   c. Athlete's foot.

   d. Barber's itch.

19. Acrochordon, common benign skin growths, may also be called:

    a. Skin tags.

    b. Actinic keratosis.

    c. Epidermal cyst.

    d. Keloids and hypertrophic scars.

20. Function(s) of the skin include:

    a. To protect the body from trauma, infections, and toxic chemicals.

    b. To synthesize vitamin D.

    c. To regulate body temperature.

    d. All of the above.

21. What is another name of an inflammatory condition of the sebaceous, or oil, glands?

    a. Atopic dermatitis.

    b. Seborrheic dermatitis.

    c. Urticarial.

    d. Rosacea.

SCENARIO

Scenario will require students to use critical thinking skills to determine the various possible answers. Some research may be necessary to include an evidence-based answer.

Parents have a 2-month-old, a 2-year-old, and a 4-year-old. The 2-month-old was diagnosed with seborrheic dermatitis or cradle cap. The parents are informed cradle cap is an inflammation of the sebaceous glands and is common in infants. The patients review video on how to shampoo, massage, and rinse the head daily with a mild shampoo. They review the written instructions including how to look for loosen, and remove scales.

1. The parents are very concerned dermatitis is 'catching'. Explain what additional information needs to be shared with the parents.

_____

_____

_____

_____

7 Diseases and Conditions of the Musculoskeletal System

WORD DEFINITIONS

Define the following basic medical terms.

1. Adjacent _____

2. Bacterium _____

3. Bunionectomy _____

4. Calcanean _____

5. Calcification _____

6. Collagen _____

7. Edematous _____

8. Extension _____

9. Fasciitis _____

10. Flexion _____

11. Hyperbaric oxygen treatment _____

12. Hyperostosis _____

13. Intraarticular _____

14. Laxity _____

15. Osteotomy _____

16. Plantar _____

GLOSSARY TERMS

Define the following chapter glossary terms.

1. Abscess _____

2. Arthrodesis _____

3. Arthroplasty _____

4. Cheilectomy _____

5. Closed reduction _____

6. Echocardiographic _____

7. Hallux _____

8. Hyperuricemia _____

9. Magnetic resonance imaging _____

10. Metatarsophalangeal _____

11. Open reduction _____

12. Osteophytes _____

13. Periosteum _____

14. Purulent _____

15. Sclerosing _____

16. Sequestrum _____

17. Skeletal traction _____

18. Subluxation _____

19. Synovial _____

20. Tendinitis _____

SHORT ANSWER

Answer the following questions.

1. List the three types of muscle tissues as defined histologically.

_____

2. Identify when shin splints are likely to occur.

_____

3. Cite the cause of fibromyalgia.

_____

4. Is there a specific laboratory test to identify whether a patient has fibromyalgia?

_____

5. Name the most common form of arthritis.

_____

6. Identify one common cause for the delay in making the correct diagnosis of Lyme Disease.

_____

7. Describe the rash that sometimes accompanies Lyme disease.

_____

_____

8. List the three types of muscle tissues as defined histologically.

_____

9. Identify the cause of gouty arthritis.

_____

10. Name the hereditary syndrome that affects the connective tissue and causes an abnormal growth of the extremities.

_____

11. Cite the other name for Paget's disease.

_____

12. Identify the most common sites of the body affected by Paget's disease.

_____

13. Name the most common type of primary bone neoplasm.

_____

14. A deficiency in vitamin D may cause what abnormal metabolic bone disease?

_____

15. Which gender is more likely to be affected by osteoporosis?

_____

16. Name the term for a benign growth filled with a jellylike substance that commonly develops on the back of the wrist and may be caused by repetitive injury.

_____

17. Cite the other name for a hallux valgus.

_____

18. Name the injury that involves the semilunar cartilages in the knee.

_____

109

19. List the three abnormal curvatures of the spine.

_____

20. Identify the structures in the skeletal system affected by osteoarthritis.

_____

21. In what state and in what year was Lyme disease first detected?

_____

22. List the classic symptoms of bursitis.

_____

23. Name the medication that may be injected into the joint to treat bursitis.

_____

24. Identify the area of the foot that is usually affected by gout.

_____

25. Name the most common metabolic bone disease characterized by loss of bone mass and density.

_____

26. What determines the prognosis for primary bone cancer?

_____

27. List the terms used to classify sprains.

_____

28. Gangrene, severe trauma, malignancy, or congenital defects are some conditions that may necessitate surgical removal of a limb. Name the procedure that is performed to accomplish this.

_____

29. Are muscle tumors often benign?

_____

30. Which area of the body is affected when a person has plantar fasciitis?

_____

31. What can a person do to prevent heel spurs?

_____

32. What diagnostic test is considered best for osteoporosis?

_____

33. How soon should a patient with traumatic dislocation be seen by a physician?

_____

FILL IN THE BLANKS

Fill in the blanks with the correct terms. A word list has been provided.

Word List

amputation, back, body, bones, bony, cardiac, cartilage, ends, facilitate, femur, ganglion, gestation, humerus, limb, movement, muscle, muscle atrophy, muscles, nonstriated, organs, osteogenesis, serotonin, striated, surface, tendons, third, tibia, tissue, vertebrae

1. All movement, including the movement of the _____ themselves and the _____, is performed by _____ tissue.

2. The three types of muscle tissue are _____ or skeletal, _____ or smooth, and _____.

3. Bones develop through a process called _____.

4. The complete skeleton is formed by the end of the _____ month of _____.

5. Joints are classified according to their _____.

6. The _____ is a semismooth, dense, supporting connective _____ that is found at the _____ of _____.

7. A patient with fibromyalgia has a relatively low level of the brain nerve chemical _____.

8. Bursae are found between _____ and _____ and cover _____ prominences, to _____ movement.

9. The most commonly involved bones in osteomyelitic infections are the upper ends of the _____ and _____, the lower end of the _____, and occasionally the _____.

10. Phantom _____ sensation is an unpleasant complication that sometimes follows a(an) _____.

11. Permanent _____ can result from tendon damage.

12. A(an) _____ most commonly develops on the _____ of the wrist as a single, smooth lump, just under the _____ of the skin.

Identify the structures of the following anatomic diagrams.

1. Normal muscular system—anterior view

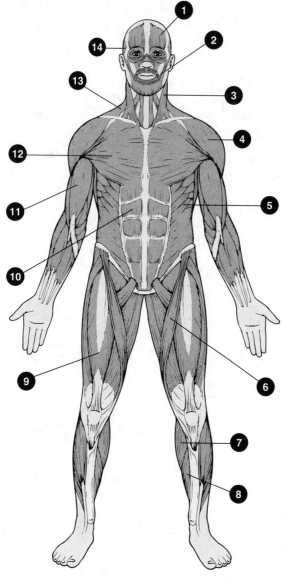

(1) _____   (8) _____

(2) _____   (9) _____

(3) _____   (10) _____

(4) _____   (11) _____

(5) _____   (12) _____

(6) _____   (13) _____

(7) _____   (14) _____

2. Normal muscular system—posterior view

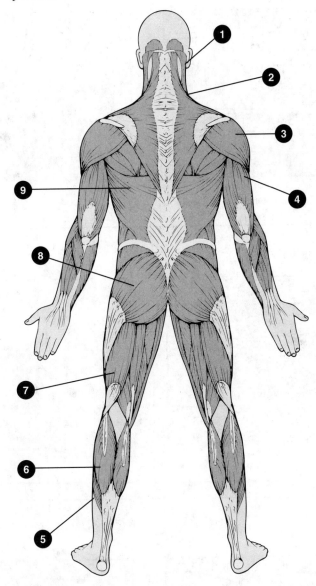

(1) _____   (6) _____

(2) _____   (7) _____

(3) _____   (8) _____

(4) _____   (9) _____

(5) _____

3. Types of muscles

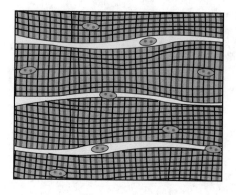 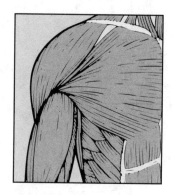

_____

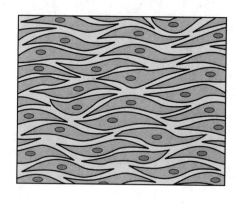 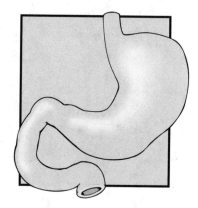

_____

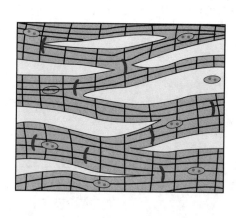 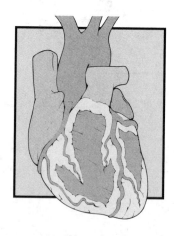

_____

114

4. Normal skeletal system—anterior view

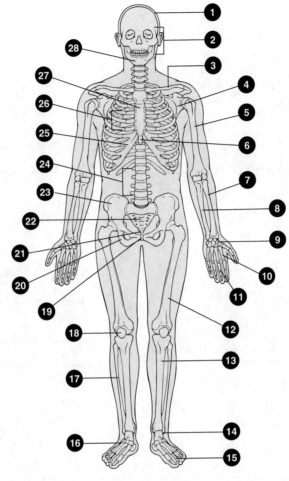

(1) _____

(2) _____

(3) _____

(4) _____

(5) _____

(6) _____

(7) _____

(8) _____

(9) _____

(10) _____

(11) _____

(12) _____

(13) _____

(14) _____

(15) _____

(16) _____

(17) _____

(18) _____

(19) _____

(20) _____

(21) _____

(22) _____

(23) _____

(24) _____

(25) _____

(26) _____

(27) _____

(28) _____

115

5. Examples of types of joints

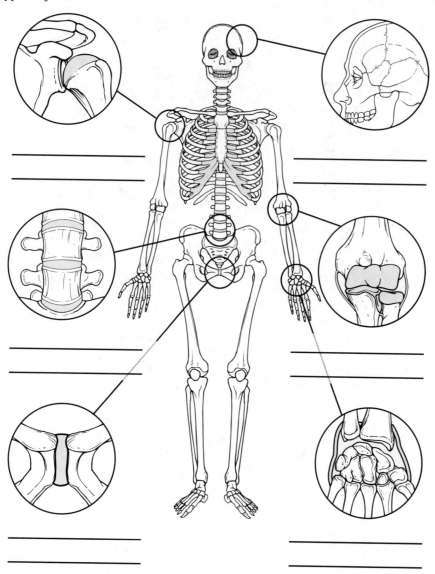

_____ _____

_____ _____

_____ _____

_____ _____

6. Types of fractures

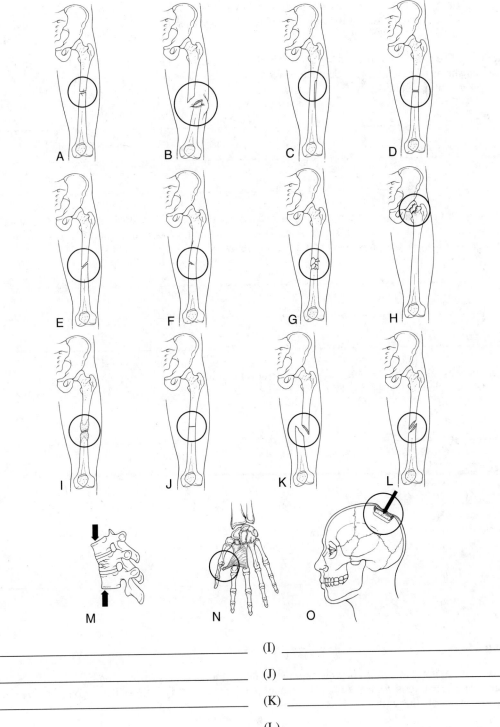

(A) _____

(B) _____

(C) _____

(D) _____

(E) _____

(F) _____

(G) _____

(H) _____

(I) _____

(J) _____

(K) _____

(L) _____

(M) _____

(N) _____

(O) _____

117

PATIENT SCREENING

For each of the following scenarios, explain how and why you would schedule an appointment or suggest a referral based on the patient's reported symptoms. First review the "Guidelines for Patient-Screening Exercises" found on p. iv in the Introduction.

1. The mother of a 12-year-old girl calls in saying that her daughter has started complaining of back pain and fatigue. She also states that she has noticed that her daughter's skirts do not hang evenly and that the school nurse has suggested an examination for scoliosis. How do you handle this phone call?

   _____

   _____

   _____

2. A patient calls asking for an appointment saying that he has a red, itchy rash with a red circle in the center resembling the bull's eye on a target (target lesion) on his arm. He tells you that he was in the woods 2 days ago and thinks that a tick bit him. He thinks that the physician should see him. How do you respond to this call?

   _____

   _____

   _____

3. A male patient calls telling you that he is experiencing severe, almost excruciating pain in the first joint of his left great toe. He has experienced this before, and the pain usually peaks after several hours and then subsides gradually. He also has a slight fever and chills. How do you respond to this call?

   _____

   _____

   _____

4. A patient calls the office saying that he just twisted his ankle while walking up the stairs. He is complaining of localized pain and says he cannot stand on his leg. How do you handle this call?

   _____

   _____

   _____

5. A patient calls in saying that, while she was cutting a watermelon, her knife slipped and she cut the middle finger on her left hand. The bleeding is controlled but she cannot bend her finger. The physician is gone from the office for the day. How do you handle this call?

   _____

   _____

   _____

PATIENT TEACHING

For each scenario below, outline the appropriate patient teaching you would perform. First review the "Guidelines for Patient-Teaching Exercises" found on p. iv in the Introduction.

1. OSTEOARTHRITIS

   An established patient with a history of osteoarthritis is undergoing ongoing therapy, which includes drug therapy and a gentle exercise regimen. The patient is discouraged because of increased pain and loss of mobility. The physician instructs you to provide printed information regarding therapeutic diets and exercise for the patient. In addition, you are to review intended effects of the prescribed drug therapy. How do you handle this patient-teaching opportunity?

   _____

   _____

   _____

   _____

2. LYME DISEASE

   A male patient has been diagnosed with Lyme disease. Antibiotic therapy has been prescribed. The patient has been told to return for a checkup in 1 week. The physician asks you to provide the patient with printed information concerning therapy that is advised in the treatment of this condition. How would you handle this patient-teaching opportunity?

   _____

   _____

   _____

   _____

3. GOUT

   An individual has been diagnosed with gout. The physician has instructed you to provide the patient with printed information regarding therapy for treatment of gout. How do you approach this patient-teaching opportunity?

   _____

   _____

   _____

4. OSTEOPOROSIS

   An older woman has been diagnosed with osteoporosis. The physician asks you to provide the patient with printed information concerning therapy that is advised in the treatment of this condition. How do you handle this patient-teaching opportunity?

   _____

   _____

   _____

   _____

5. FRACTURES

An individual has a fracture of the ulna and radius at the wrist. A cast was placed on the area a few weeks earlier, and the patient is now requesting additional information about therapy for the hand, wrist, and arm. The physician has explained the anticipated therapy to the patient and asks you to review this information with him or her. How do you handle this patient-teaching opportunity?

_____

_____

_____

_____

PHARMACOLOGY QUESTIONS

Circle the letter of the choice that best completes the statement or answers the question.

1. Which of the following medications is classified as a muscle relaxant?

   a. Celecoxib (Celebrex)

   b. Ibuprofen (Motrin)

   c. Cyclobenzaprine (Flexeril)

   d. Colchicine

2. Treatment of fibromyalgia may include all of the following except:

   a. Naproxen (Naprosyn).

   b. Amitriptyline (Elavil).

   c. Alendronate (Fosamax).

   d. Oxaprozin (Daypro).

3. Which of the following antiinflammatory drugs has been reported to have less gastrointestinal irritation?

   a. Indomethacin (Indocin)

   b. Celecoxib (Celebrex)

   c. Naproxen (Naprosyn)

   d. Oxaprozin (Daypro)

4. Bursitis is commonly treated with the following except for:

   a. Application of moist heat.

   b. Nonsteroidal antiinflammatory drugs.

   c. Corticosteroid drugs.

   d. Muscle relaxants.

5. Treatment of gout may include which of the following?

   a. Colchicine

   b. Dietary modifications

   c. Corticosteroids

   d. All of the above

120

6. Prevention of bone loss and osteoporosis is attempted by the use of the following drugs, except for:

   a. Alendronate (Fosamax).

   b. Risedronate (Actonel).

   c. Calcitonin salmon (Miacalcin).

   d. Tizanidine (Zanaflex).

7. In the process of bone formation, which vitamin is necessary for the absorption of calcium and phosphorus?

   a. Vitamin D

   b. Vitamin B_6

   c. Vitamin C

   d. None of the above

8. Which medication could be used to treat the inflammation from bunions?

   a. Sildenafil (Viagra)

   b. Sulfasalazine (Azulfidine)

   c. Phenazopyridine (Pyridium)

   d. Indomethacin (Indocin)

9. Shin splints are often treated with rest, application of ice or heat, and:

   a. Gradual physical therapy.

   b. Antiinflammatory drugs.

   c. Specific stretching exercises.

   d. All of the above.

10. Drug therapy for osteoarthritis can include:

    a. Analgesics.

    b. NSAIDs.

    c. Muscle relaxants.

    d. All of the above.

ESSAY QUESTION

Write a response to the following question or statement. Use a separate sheet of paper if more space is needed.

1. Describe the possible treatments for simple and compound fractures.

_____

_____

_____

_____

_____

_____

_____

_____

_____

_____

_____

_____

2. If osteoporosis is not diagnosed and treated, what complications may develop?

_____

_____

_____

3. Explain tendons and their importance in the musculoskeletal system.

_____

_____

_____

4. Define the primary objectives of the treatment for Lorodosis caused by pregnancy and obesity and what can be the results if untreated.

_____

_____

_____

_____

5. What other systems may be affected if the patient with scoliosis does not seek treatment?

_____

_____

_____

6. Osteoarthritis cannot be cured, so the goal of treatment is to reduce inflammation, minimize pain, and maintain functioning joints. Describe the following treatments

Drug therapy: _____

_____

Nutritional management: _____

_____

Supportive care: _____

_____

Surgery: _____

_____

7. Explain the processes called osteogenesis and ossification in bone development.

_____

_____

_____

_____

Circle the letter of the choice that best completes the statement or answers the question.

1. Lordosis is a(an) _____ curvature of the spine.

    a. Lateral

    b. Inward (swayback)

    c. Outward

    d. None of the above

2. Scoliosis is a(an) _____ curvature of the spine.

    a. Lateral

    b. Inward (swayback)

    c. Outward

    d. None of the above

3. Kyphosis is a(an) _____ curvature of the spine.

    a. Lateral

    b. Inward (swayback)

    c. Outward

    d. None of the above

4. Gouty arthritis is an inflammation of the joints caused by:

    a. An excessive level of uric acid in the joints.

    b. An excessive level of serum protein.

    c. Streptococcus bacteria.

    d. None of the above.

5. A fracture with a break in the bone and a wound is a _____ fracture.

    a. Spiral

    b. Comminuted

    c. Compound, through the skin

    d. None of the above

6. A fracture with splintered or crushed bone is a _____ fracture.

    a. Comminuted

    b. Simple

    c. Greenstick

    d. None of the above

7. When a bone is fractured as a result of disease, it is called a _____ fracture.

    a. Greenstick

    b. Pathologic

    c. Spiral

    d. None of the above

8. An inflammatory response at the bottom of the heel bone is called:

    a. Plantar fasciitis.

    b. Calcaneal spur.

    c. Both a and b.

    d. None of the above.

9. A severed tendon causes immediate and severe pain, inflammation, and:

    a. Decreased mobility of the affected part.

    b. Complete immobility of the affected part.

    c. Weakness of the affected part.

    d. None of the above.

10. Spurs are a common problem diagnosed in:

    a. Individuals with bone deficiency.

    b. Individuals active in sports, especially runners.

    c. Individuals who use repetitive hand and wrist motions in their employment.

    d. None of the above.

11. Lyme disease is transmitted from a bacterium that is carried by a:

    a. Mosquito.

    b. Bee.

    c. Tick.

    d. All of the above.

12. Tendons are tough strands or cords of dense connective tissue that attach muscle to:

    a. Muscle.

    b. Joints.

    c. Bones.

    d. None of the above.

13. Collagen is a major supporting element or glue in:

    a. Muscles.

    b. Ligaments.

    c. Connective tissue.

    d. None of the above.

125

14. The skeletal system is composed of _____ bones.

    a. 200

    b. 208

    c. 308

    d. None of the above

15. Osteomyelitis is a(an):

    a. Chronic progressive inflammatory disease.

    b. Infection in a bone that can lead to abscess formation and sequestrum when not properly cared for.

    c. Progressive weakening of the skeletal muscles.

    d. None of the above.

16. Adhesive capsulitis (frozen shoulder):

    a. Can result in permanent impairment of mobility of the shoulder.

    b. Occurs more frequently in patients with diabetes.

    c. Usually begins after an injury or a case of bursitis or tendinitis.

    d. All of the above.

17. Symptoms and signs of bone tumors may include:

    a. Pain.

    b. No pain.

    c. A limp.

    d. All of the above.

18. Treatment of Lyme disease:

    a. Begins with removal of the tick.

    b. Requires early antibiotic therapy for a cure.

    c. If delayed, can result in damage to joints, heart, or nervous system.

    d. All of the above.

19. Paget's disease (osteitis deformans) is a chronic bone disorder that results in:

    a. Stronger bones.

    b. Enlarged, deformed, weakened bones.

    c. Severe symptoms for all patients with the disease.

    d. None of the above.

20. Marfan syndrome is a group of inherited conditions featuring:

    a. Abnormally long extremities and digits.

    b. Abnormal connective tissues.

    c. Weakness of blood vessels.

    d. All of the above.

21. Bone tumors, whether benign or malignant, are treated by:

    a. Surgical excision.

    b. Radiation.

    c. Chemotherapy.

    d. Weight-bearing exercise.

22. In adults, osteomalacia causes bones to become increasingly:

    a. Soft.

    b. Flexible.

    c. Deformed.

    d. All of the above.

23. One of the most common chronic diseases affecting the muscles and soft tissue surrounding the joint is:

    a. Fibromyalgia.

    b. Plantar fasciitis.

    c. Lordosis.

    d. None of the above.

24. Collapse of thoracic vertebrae from the weakened bone of osteoporosis is often responsible for the "hunchback" in the older person and is called:

    a. Hallux Rigidus.

    b. Gout.

    c. Dowager's Hump.

    d. Ganglion.

25. Which statement is true about osteomyelitis?

    a. It is a self-limiting condition.

    b. It is caused by chronic poor posture.

    c. It is a serious infection of bone.

    d. It is usually cured by rest and increased fluid intake.

26. Which of the following statements is(are) true about osteosarcoma?

    a. The tumor weakens the bone, making it prone to fracture.

    b. It is treated by surgical incision.

    c. It often metastasizes to the lungs.

    d. All of the above.

Critical Thinking: What is the understanding of the muscle classified as either voluntary or involuntary?

_____

_____

_____

_____

_____

Scenario

A patient is diagnosed with plantar fasciitis. She is in the office for the second time in 2 weeks.

QUESTIONS:

a. The patient asks you why she is not better?

_____

_____

_____

_____

_____

b. What information about plantar fasciitis should be given to her?

_____

_____

_____

_____

_____

8 Diseases and Conditions of the Digestive System

WORD DEFINITIONS

Define the following basic medical terms.

1. Apicectomy _____

2. Cholinergic _____

3. Colectomy _____

4. Erosion _____

5. Fissure _____

6. Fistula _____

7. Gangrene _____

8. Hematemesis _____

9. Leukoplakia _____

10. Ligation _____

11. Lymphadenopathy _____

12. Malaise _____

13. Metastasis _____

14. Odynophagia _____

15. Pseudomembranous _____

16. Retrosternal _____

17. Valsalva's maneuver _____

GLOSSARY TERMS

Define the following chapter glossary terms.

1. Anastomoses _____

2. Aphthous ulcers _____

3. Cachexia _____

4. Diaphoretic _____

5. Fissures _____

6. Fistulas _____

7. Gangrene _____

8. H$_2$-receptor antagonist _____

9. Hemostasis _____

10. Hepatomegaly _____

11. Hyperemic _____

12. Hypovolemic shock _____

13. Jaundiced _____

14. Lavage _____

15. Malocclusion _____

16. Myalgia _____

17. Peritonitis _____

18. Proton pump inhibitor _____

19. Reflux _____

20. Steatorrhea _____

21. Odynophagia _____

22. Tenesmus _____

23. Xerostomia _____

SHORT ANSWER

Answer the following questions.

1. Identify the function of the teeth.

_____

2. List four main reasons that a person may be missing permanent teeth.

_____

_____

3. Describe how oral tumors begin.

_____

4. What symptom usually prompts a person to seek medical treatment for temporomandibular joint syndrome?

_____

5. Is thrush a bacterial, fungal, or viral infection?

_____

6. Cite statistics of incidence of squamous cell oral cancers.

_____

7. What lifestyle factors contribute to up to 80% of cases of oral cancer?

_____

_____

8. List treatment options for oral cancer.

_____

9. Identify the main symptom that a patient experiences with esophagitis.

_____

10. Name the main cause of gastritis.

_____

11. Name the country with the highest incidence of gastric cancer in the world.

_____

12. Name one of the most severe consequences of chronic gastroesophageal reflux disease.

_____

13. Cite the length of the appendix.

_____

14. Identify the function of the appendix.

_____

15. Name the device that patients sometimes wear if they have a hernia.

_____

16. Identify the area of the alimentary canal that can be affected by Crohn's disease.

_____

17. Name the type of cancer that a patient with chronic ulcerative colitis is at risk to develop.

_____

18. Explain the goal of treatment for gastroenteritis.

_____

_____

19. List the symptoms and signs of intestinal obstruction.

_____

20. Which part of the colon is usually the site of diverticulosis?

_____

21. Name the third most common site of cancer incidence and cause of death in both men and women.

_____

22. At what age should annual fecal occult testing begin for people at average risk for colorectal cancer?

_____

23. Can peritonitis be life threatening?

_____

24. In which gender is cirrhosis diagnosed more frequently?

_____

25. Identify the incubation period for hepatitis A.

_____

26. List the four fat-soluble vitamins that are stored in fat tissue.

_____

27. What is biofilm?

_____

28. Name the peptic ulcer that is most common and located in the first part of the small intestine.

_____

29. Can peptic ulcers be healed?

_____

30. What eating disorder is one of the most difficult to treat?

_____

FILL IN THE BLANKS

Fill in the blanks with the correct terms. A word list has been provided.

Word List

absorb, alimentary canal, anal canal, base, bland diet, contagious, damage, days, digestion, disease, easily, esophageal, fails, gluten intolerance, gum, hiatal, hematemesis, inflammation, insufficient, lips, malabsorption, mastication, mouth, oral, overeating, periodontal, recovery, shock, small intestine, sterile, stomach, strong, swallowed, syndrome, teeth, tissue, tooth abscess, transparent, ulcers, upper, varicose, vitamins, volvulus, weight, white

1. The _____ processes and transports products of _____.

2. The function of the teeth is _____ to break down food into pieces that can be _____ and digested _____.

3. Periodontitis, also called _____ disease, is destructive _____ and bone _____ around one or more of the _____.

4. A _____ is a pus-filled sac that develops in the _____ surrounding the _____ of the root.

5. Herpes simplex blisters can develop on the _____ and inside the _____, producing painful _____ that last a few hours or _____.

6. Oral cancer usually appears as a(an) _____, patchy lesion, or a(an) _____ ulcer that _____ to heal.

7. Esophageal reflux can result from _____, pregnancy, or _____ gain, and other causes as well.

8. Treatment of mild esophagitis includes several weeks of a(an) _____ to calm the _____ and the use of _____ antacids.

9. A _____ hernia exists when the _____ part of the _____ protrudes through the _____ opening of the diaphragm into the thoracic cavity.

10. A _____ is a mechanical bowel obstruction in which there is a twisting of the bowel on itself.

11. Short-bowel _____ is the result of a(an) _____ amount of functioning small bowel to _____ nutrients, fluid, _____, and minerals that the body needs.

12. Hemorrhoids are _____ dilations of a vein in the _____ or the anorectal area.

13. Viral hepatitis is _____ until _____ is complete.

14. Celiac disease is a disease of the _____ that is characterized by _____, _____, and _____ to the lining of the intestine.

15. When esophageal varices rupture, the patient experiences _____ and signs of hypovolemic _____.

16. Peritonitis, the inflammation of the peritoneum, can be acute or chronic and local or generalized. The large serous membrane that lines the abdominal cavity and folds over the visceral organs is normally _____ and _____.

ANATOMIC STRUCTURES

Identify the following structures of the digestive system and their functions.

1. Main and accessory organs of the normal digestive system

Accessory Organs   **Main Organs**

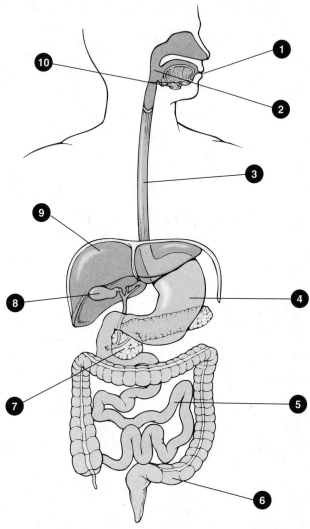

(1) _____

(2) _____

(3) _____

(4) _____

(5) _____

(6) _____

(7) _____

(8) _____

(9) _____

(10) _____

134

PATIENT SCREENING

For each of the following scenarios, explain how and why you would schedule an appointment or suggest a referral based on the patient's reported symptoms. First review the "Guidelines for Patient-Screening Exercises" found on p. iv in the Introduction.

1. A male patient calls stating that he is experiencing pain in the "jaw joint" on the right side of his mouth. He says that he has been hearing a clicking sound when he chews and the pain is getting progressively worse. He also says that he is having problems opening his mouth. He requests an appointment to see the physician. How do you handle this phone call?

   _____

   _____

   _____

2. A patient calls stating that he is experiencing "heartburn," usually most severe at night. He also says that he has episodes of belching, causing a burning sensation in his mouth and chest. How do you handle this phone call?

   _____

   _____

   _____

3. The father of a 16-year-old adolescent calls the office stating that his son is experiencing abdominal pain that started as vague discomfort around the navel. Now a few hours later it has localized in the right lower quadrant. He has just become nauseated and has a slight fever. How do you handle this call?

   _____

   _____

   _____

4. A patient calls stating that she is experiencing pain in the right upper quadrant of the abdomen, often radiating to the right upper back in the area of the scapula. Nausea and vomiting accompany the pain. She thinks that her skin is turning yellow. How do you respond to this call?

   _____

   _____

   _____

5. The mother of a 16-year-old adolescent calls advising that she wants her daughter to be seen by the physician. The girl is refusing to eat and is preoccupied with obesity and obsessed with her weight. Although she experiences continued weight loss, she does not believe that anything is wrong. How do you handle this phone call?

   _____

   _____

   _____

PATIENT TEACHING

For each of the following scenarios, outline the appropriate patient teaching you would perform. First review the "Guidelines for Patient-Teaching Exercises" found on p. iv in the Introduction.

1. DENTAL CARIES

   A patient is noted to be in need of dental assessment. The physician suggests that, until a dental appointment can be made and kept, the patient should be instructed on proper oral hygiene and dental care. How do you handle this patient-teaching opportunity?

   _____

   _____

   _____

   _____

   _____

2. HERPES SIMPLEX

   A patient has a large "cold sore" on the upper lip that is quite painful. It is diagnosed as a herpes simplex eruption. You are instructed to provide printed information regarding the care of the eruption and ways to prevent spreading this contagious lesion. How do you approach this patient-teaching opportunity?

   _____

   _____

   _____

   _____

   _____

3. GASTROESOPHAGEAL REFLUX DISORDER

   An individual experiencing gastroesophageal reflux disorder (GERD) requires instructions about methods to prevent the reflux. The physician asks you to provide him or her with printed information and explain how he or she can lessen the occurrence of the attacks. How do you approach this patient-teaching opportunity?

   _____

   _____

   _____

   _____

   _____

4. PEPTIC ULCERS

An individual has been diagnosed with a peptic ulcer. The physician asks that you reinforce his instructions to the patient by using printed material available in the office. How do you approach this patient-teaching opportunity?

_____

_____

_____

_____

_____

_____

5. CHOLECYSTITIS

An individual has been experiencing severe right-sided epigastric pain after eating. The diagnosis of cholecystitis has been made. The physician asks you to reinforce her dietary instructions to the patient using printed dietary information available in the office. How do you approach this patient-teaching opportunity?

_____

_____

_____

_____

_____

_____

_____

PHARMACOLOGY QUESTIONS

Circle the letter of the choice that best completes the statement or answers the question.

1. Some medications may cause discoloration of the teeth. Which of the following drugs has been shown to discolor teeth when taken during early childhood?

    a. Penicillin

    b. Sulfamethoxazole

    c. Tetracycline

    d. Prednisone

2. In advanced cases of gingivitis, which antibacterial mouthwash is frequently prescribed?

    a. Lugol's solution

    b. Listerine

    c. 0.9% sodium chloride

    d. Chlorhexidine (Periogard)

3. Oral thrush *(Candida albicans)* is often treated with which oral antifungal agent?

   a. Cephalexin (Keflex)

   b. Atorvastatin (Lipitor)

   c. Nystatin

   d. Simvastatin (Zocor)

4. GERD may be treated with all of the following except:

   a. Theophylline.

   b. Omeprazole (Prilosec).

   c. A decrease in cigarette smoking.

   d. Elevation of the head of the bed.

5. Which of the following drugs should be avoided in a patient with a peptic ulcer?

   a. Esomeprazole (Nexium)

   b. Naproxen sodium (Aleve)

   c. Ranitidine (Zantac)

   d. Cimetidine (Tagamet)

6. Which of the following is used to treat peptic ulcers?

   a. Lansoprazole (Prevacid)

   b. Pregabalin (Lyrica)

   c. Metformin (Glucophage)

   d. Glimepiride (Amaryl)

7. The treatment of ulcerative colitis may include all of the following except:

   a. Corticosteroids.

   b. Sulfasalazine (Azulfidine).

   c. Timolol (Timoptic).

   d. Anticholinergic agents.

8. Inflammation of the peritoneum (peritonitis) may be treated with any or all of the following except:

   a. Methylphenidate (Ritalin).

   b. Broad-spectrum antibiotics.

   c. Parenteral electrolytes.

   d. Pain killers.

9. Which of the following medications may be used to treat motion sickness?

   a. Cimetidine (Tagamet)

   b. Dimenhydrinate (Dramamine)

   c. Metoclopramide (Reglan)

   d. Omeprazole (Prilosec)

Write a response to the following question or statement. Use a separate sheet of paper if more space is needed.

1. Describe the signs and symptoms that are associated with Crohn's disease and available options for treatment.

_____

_____

_____

_____

_____

_____

_____

_____

_____

_____

_____

_____

_____

2. Describe patient screening for a hiatal hernia.

_____

_____

_____

_____

3. Discuss the cause of gastroenteritis.

_____

_____

_____

_____

4. Explain the function of the small intestine.

_____

_____

_____

_____

5. Define the prognosis for peptic ulcers.

_____

_____

_____

_____

6. What other complications could the patient with acute appendicitis experience if they do not seek treatment?

_____

_____

_____

_____

7. List the three criteria needed for a positive diagnosis of celiac disease.

_____

_____

_____

_____

8. Discuss the relationship between anorexia and bulimia.

_____

_____

_____

_____

_____

_____

Circle the letter of the choice that best completes the statement or answers the question.

1. The transmission route for _____ is fecal-oral and is transmitted by contaminated water, food, and stools. Poor hygiene also plays a role in the transmission.

    a. Hepatitis A

    b. Hepatitis B

    c. Hepatitis C

    d. None of the above

2. The use of broad-spectrum antibiotics is associated with the occurrence of:

    a. Esophagitis.

    b. Gastritis.

    c. Pseudomembranous enterocolitis.

    d. None of the above.

3. The symptoms of biliary colic with radiating pain and jaundice accompany:

    a. Appendicitis.

    b. Cholecystitis.

    c. Cholelithiasis.

    d. Both b and c.

4. Anorexia nervosa is an eating disorder in which the person perceives his or her body image as:

    a. Thin.

    b. Just right.

    c. Overweight.

    d. None of the above.

5. A chronic irreversible degeneration of the liver is:

    a. Cholecystitis.

    b. Pancreatitis.

    c. Cholelithiasis.

    d. Cirrhosis.

6. The route of transmission for _____ is by blood or body fluid.

    a. Hepatitis A

    b. Hepatitis B

    c. Hepatitis C

    d. Both b and c

7. Peritonitis is an infection that involves the:

    a. Liver.

    b. Serous membrane that lines the abdominal cavity.

c. Pancreas.

d. None of the above.

8. Neoplasm, volvulus, intussusception, and fecal impaction can all cause:

a. Diverticulitis.

b. Diverticulosis.

c. Mechanical bowel obstruction.

d. None of the above.

9. The fourth leading cause of cancer-related death in the United States is:

a. Colon cancer.

b. Gastric cancer.

c. Pancreatic cancer.

d. None of the above.

10. Allergic reaction or irritation from foods, mechanical injury, medications, poisons, alcohol, and infectious diseases may damage the gastric lining and cause:

a. Diverticulitis.

b. Gastritis.

c. Hepatitis.

d. None of the above.

11. The following statements about periodontitis are true, except:

a. The cause is plaque biofilm.

b. It is not related to gingivitis.

c. Early detection and treatment can help prevent tooth loss.

d. Chemotherapy, diabetes, smoking, and HIV are contributing factors.

12. The clinical management of Barrett's esophagus includes:

a. Treatment of the symptoms of GERD.

b. Endoscopic surveillance every 3 years to detect dysplasia.

c. Acid-suppressive medications, lifestyle changes, and possibly antireflux surgery.

d. All of the above.

13. Pseudomembranous enterocolitis, an infection with *Clostridum difficile*, is common in health care facilities. Prevention measures include:

a. Drugs that slow bowel activity.

b. Use of alcohol-based antibacterial foams.

c. Starting a broad-spectrum antibiotic.

d. None of the above.

14. Hiatal hernia is the condition in which:

    a. The patient reports heartburn that is worse on reclining or after a large meal.

    b. The cause is functional rather than organic.

    c. Respiratory complications such as aspiration or asthma can develop.

    d. Both a and c.

15. The diagnosis of irritable bowel syndrome:

    a. Is based largely on abnormal laboratory findings.

    b. Excludes organic disease.

    c. Involves normal gastrointestinal motility.

    d. All of the above.

16. Which disease has a higher morbidity and mortality rate than any other source of gastrointestinal bleeding?

    a. Bleeding esophageal varices

    b. Diverticulitis

    c. Hiatal hernia

    d. Hemorrhoids

17. The diagnostic test for esophagitis that is considered a superior method and includes biopsy is called:

    a. Liver function study.

    b. Esophagoscopy.

    c. A chest film.

    d. A barium study.

18. Patients with Barrett's esophagus usually undergo endoscopies to screen for progression to:

    a. Adenocarcinoma.

    b. Osteosarcoma.

    c. Both of the above.

    d. None of the above.

19. Which statement is true about food poisoning?

    a. Symptoms are not related to the cause.

    b. Infection control is the first line of defense.

    c. Food poisoning is always self-limiting.

    d. None of the above are true.

20. Overweight and obesity are identified objectively by:

    a. Gender, race, and weight.

    b. Age, ethnicity, and weight.

    c. Use of the body mass index (BMI).

    d. All of the above.

143

21. What are the three accessory organs of digestion that introduce digestive hormones and enzymes into the alimentary canal, ensuring that the nutrients critical to life can be absorbed selectively by the small intestines into the bloodstream?

   a. Pancreas, duodenum, and gallbladder

   b. Stomach, small intestines, and diaphragm

   c. Colon, pancreas, and liver

   d. Liver, gallbladder, and pancreas

22. What disease can mimic appendicitis, requiring prompt medical investigation?

   a. Abdominal Hernia

   b. Gastritis

   c. Crohn Disease

   d. Hiatal Hernia

SCENARIO

Scenario will require students to use critical thinking skills to determine the various possible answers. Some research may be necessary to include an evidence-based answer.

A new mother is breastfeeding and notices white patches on the infant's tongue and sides of the mouth. The mother does not know what is happening and seeks medical attention to determine what is wrong. After the examination, the mother is informed the diagnosis is thrush. She is given a prescription and an opportunity to ask questions. Instead, the mother begins to cry and believes the thrush is her fault.

Explain what thrush is, the etiology, frequency, and usual treatment.

_____

_____

_____

_____

_____

b. What other information could be shared with the new mother?

_____

_____

_____

_____

_____

9 Diseases and Conditions of the Respiratory System

WORD DEFINITIONS

Define the following basic medical terms.

1. Auscultation _____

2. Dysphagia _____

3. Hepatomegaly _____

4. Hypercapnia _____

5. Hypocapnia _____

6. Laryngectomy _____

7. Mucopurulent _____

8. Myalgia _____

9. Opacities _____

10. Purulent _____

11. Rhinitis _____

12. Sclerosing _____

13. Suprasternal _____

14. Tinnitus _____

15. Venostasis _____

GLOSSARY TERMS

Define the following chapter glossary terms.

1. Agranulocytosis _____

2. Aphonia _____

3. Bifurcates _____

4. Cephalgia _____

5. Coagulation _____

6. Cyanosis _____

7. Emboli _____

8. Epistaxis _____

9. Exsanguination _____

10. Insidious _____

11. Mediastinum _____

12. Mycoplasma _____

13. Perfusion _____

14. Rales _____

15. Rhonchi _____

16. Stenosis _____

17. Stridor _____

18. Substernal retraction _____

19. Tachypnea _____

20. Thoracostomy _____

SHORT ANSWER

Answer the following questions.

1. Name the primary function of the lungs.

   _____

2. Identify the dome-shaped muscle that assists with respiration.

   _____

3. Name two causes for respiratory failure.

   _____

4. Does an antibiotic effectively treat a common cold?

   _____

5. Identify the most common causes of sinusitis.

   _____

6. What is the prognosis for emphysema?

   _____

7. Name the most common cause of cancer death worldwide for both men and women.

_____

8. What condition of the upper gastrointestinal tract can result in laryngitis?

_____

9. Do nasal polyps tend to recur after surgical removal?

_____

10. When is a nosebleed considered an emergency?

_____

11. Identify the most common symptom of laryngeal neoplasms.

_____

12. Identify what occurs when a clot of foreign material lodges in and occludes an artery in pulmonary circulation.

_____

13. Where do the vast majority of pulmonary emboli originate?

_____

14. Identify the age groups at most risk for respiratory syncytial viral infection.

_____

15. Where is the causative agent of histoplasmosis found?

_____

16. What does the term *pneumoconiosis* mean?

_____

17. Name the condition that causes sharp needlelike pain and increases with inspiration and coughing.

_____

18. Identify the two types of pleurisy.

_____

19. What accumulates in the pleural cavity when hemothorax is the diagnosis?

_____

20. Describe the fracture that occurs when the patient is diagnosed with flail chest.

_____

21. Identify the intradermal test that is used to detect the presence of tuberculin antibodies.

_____

22. Is the prognosis for adult respiratory distress syndrome (ARDS) good or guarded?

_____

23. Name the primary risk factor for developing lung cancer.

_____

24. From 1982 through 1985, what contributed to the increase of tuberculosis in the United States?

_____

25. Which patients are considered at high risk for aspiration pneumonia?

_____

26. Identify the cause of a deviated septum.

_____

FILL IN THE BLANKS

Fill in the blanks with the correct terms. A word list has been provided. Words used twice are indicated with a (2).

Word List

4, 5, air, airless, behind, blood pressure, breath, breathing, bronchitis, carbon dioxide, cavities, chest pain, collapsed, contracts, drainage, epistaxis, exchanged, external, infections, inhalation, interferes, lower, lymphadenopathy, narrow, nucleus, otitis media, out, oxygen, predisposes, poor, pulmonary, relaxes, repeated damage, respiration (2), shallow, shortness, speech, sucked into, sudden, thoracostomy, tubercle bacillus, upward, winter

1. In the lungs _____ inhaled from the air is _____ with _____ from the blood; this process is called _____ respiration.

2. On inspiration the diaphragm _____, pulling downward and causing air to be _____ the lungs. During expiration the diaphragm _____, pushing _____ and forcing air _____ of the lungs.

3. An ordinary cold should clear up in _____ to _____ days.

4. General _____ health _____ one to the common cold.

5. The sinuses, _____ in the bones lying _____ the nose, are normally _____ filled.

6. Because the opening of the larynx is _____, inflammation of the larynx sometimes _____ with _____.

7. Hemorrhage from the nose, known as _____, is a common _____ emergency.

8. The larynx plays an important role in _____, swallowing, _____, and protection of the _____ airway.

9. Bronchiectasis may be caused by _____ to the bronchial wall caused by recurrent airway _____.

10. Atelectasis is a(an) _____ or _____ state of _____ tissue.

11. Respiratory syncytial virus has the greatest occurrence during the _____ months.

12. Possible complications of influenza are _____, sinusitis, _____, and cervical _____.

13. Collapse of a lung causes severe _____ of _____, sudden sharp _____, falling _____, rapid pulse, and _____ weak _____.

14. The treatment for hemothorax includes reexpanding the lung, usually by _____ with closed _____ to evacuate the blood.

15. Pulmonary tuberculosis is acquired by the _____ of a dried droplet _____ that contains the _____ _____.

ANATOMIC STRUCTURES

Identify the structures in the following anatomic diagrams.

1. Normal lower respiratory system

(1) _____   (7) _____

(2) _____   (8) _____

(3) _____   (9) _____

(4) _____   (10) _____

(5) _____   (11) _____

(6) _____   (12) _____

2. Normal upper respiratory system

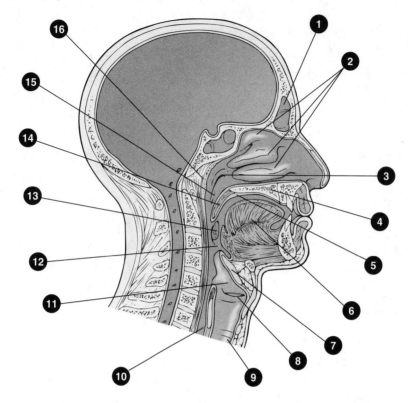

(1) _____

(2) _____

(3) _____

(4) _____

(5) _____

(6) _____

(7) _____

(8) _____

(9) _____

(10) _____

(11) _____

(12) _____

(13) _____

(14) _____

(15) _____

(16) _____

PATIENT SCREENING

For each of the following scenarios, explain how and why you would schedule an appointment or suggest a referral based on the patient's reported symptoms. First review the "Guidelines for Patient-Screening Exercises" found on p. iv in the Introduction.

1. A male patient calls to report that he is experiencing headache over both eyes, especially on waking up in the morning. He also says that there is pain and tenderness above the eyes, which occurs when bending over. In addition, he reports a thick, greenish-yellow drainage and has a slight temperature. How do you handle this phone call?

_____

_____

_____

_____

_____

2. A female patient calls saying that she is experiencing hoarseness, difficulty talking, a slight fever, and a sore throat. How do you respond to this call?

_____

_____

_____

_____

_____

3. A wife phones the office stating that her husband is experiencing a severe nosebleed. The nose has been bleeding for about 20 minutes, and they cannot get it to stop. How do you handle this phone call?

_____

_____

_____

_____

4. A male patient calls saying that he is coughing and spitting up blood. How do you respond to this call?

_____

_____

_____

_____

5. A female patient calls and advises that she is experiencing a deep, persistent, productive cough. She has thick, yellow-to-gray sputum. In addition, she reports shortness of breath; wheezing; a slightly elevated temperature; and pain in the upper chest, which is aggravated by the cough. How do you respond to this call?

_____

_____

_____

_____

PATIENT TEACHING

For each of the following scenarios, outline the appropriate patient teaching you would perform. First, review the "Guidelines for Patient-Teaching Exercises" found on p. iv in the Introduction.

1. PHARYNGITIS
   A patient has been diagnosed with recurrent pharyngitis. A course of antibiotic therapy has been prescribed. The physician has printed information regarding comfort measures. You are asked to provide the patient with the list and encourage compliance with completing the antibiotic regimen. How do you approach this patient-teaching opportunity?

_____

_____

_____

_____

2. LARYNGITIS
   Recurring laryngitis has been diagnosed for a patient who can hardly speak. The physician instructs you to explain the importance of completing the antibiotic regimen. The office has printed instructions for the patient, and you are expected to provide him or her with the list and explain any areas not fully understood. How do you approach this patient-teaching opportunity?

_____

_____

_____

_____

3. EPISTAXIS

A child has experienced recurring nosebleeds in the past few months. The parents are becoming apprehensive about them, and the physician asks you to reinforce his instructions to the parents by providing them with written information concerning epistaxis. How do you approach this patient-teaching opportunity?

_____

_____

_____

_____

_____

4. PNEUMOCONIOSIS

A patient has been diagnosed with pneumoconiosis. Along with the use of corticosteroid drugs, treatment is to include bronchodilators, oxygen therapy, and chest physical therapy to help remove secretions. How do you approach this patient-teaching opportunity?

_____

_____

_____

_____

_____

5. INFLUENZA

An individual is experiencing flulike symptoms. After being seen by the physician, the patient is diagnosed with influenza. The physician asks you to provide the patient with the printed patient-teaching instructions. How do you approach this patient-teaching opportunity?

_____

_____

_____

_____

_____

PHARMACOLOGY QUESTIONS

Circle the letter of the choice that best completes the statement or answers the question.

1. Treatment of a common cold of a viral nature could include all of the following except:

   a. Fexofenadine (Allegra).

   b. Aspirin therapy for infants and children.

   c. Acetaminophen (Tylenol).

   d. Use of a vaporizer.

2. When sinusitis or pharyngitis is of a bacterial nature, which medication is considered proper treatment?

    a. Acyclovir (Zovirax)

    b. Oseltamivir (Tamiflu)

    c. Cephalexin (Keflex)

    d. None of the above

3. Treatment of pneumonia may include all of the following except:

    a. Ciprofloxacin (Cipro).

    b. Tetracycline.

    c. Acetaminophen (Tylenol).

    d. Dicyclomine (Bentyl).

4. Influenza can be treated with which therapies?

    a. Bed rest

    b. Increased fluid intake

    c. Oseltamivir (Tamiflu)

    d. All of the above

5. Pulmonary emphysema can be treated with various therapies. Which treatment is not indicated for this diagnosis?

    a. Albuterol inhalation

    b. Ipratropium inhalation

    c. Furosemide (Lasix)

    d. Prednisone

6. Pleurisy is an inflammation of the membranes that surround the lungs. Which combination of medications would be the best therapy?

    a. Antibiotics and diuretics

    b. Antiinflammatories and beta blockers

    c. Antibiotics and beta blockers

    d. Antibiotics and analgesics

7. Infectious mononucleosis can be treated with all of the following therapies, except:

    a. Salmeterol inhaler (Serevent).

    b. Bed rest.

    c. Adequate fluid intake.

    d. Antipyretic medication.

ESSAY QUESTION

Write a response to the following question or statement. Use a separate sheet of paper if more space is needed.

1. Compare the incidence of nasopharyngeal carcinoma in males and females.

_____

_____

_____

_____

_____

2. What are the preventative measures for laryngeal cancer?

_____

_____

_____

3. Explain the way respiratory syncytial virus pneumonia is transmitted in adults.

_____

_____

_____

_____

4. Describe the major metabolic function of the lungs and kidneys in the respiratory system.

_____

_____

_____

_____

5. What is the cause of reflux laryngitis?

_____

_____

_____

_____

155

6. What is the function of the alveoli?

_____

_____

_____

_____

7. Why are the common causes of nosebleeds?

_____

_____

_____

_____

8. Discuss the importance of identifying patients with infectious tuberculosis, including measures of treatment.

_____

_____

_____

_____

_____

CERTIFICATION EXAMINATION REVIEW

Circle the letter of the choice that best completes the statement or answers the question.

1. Dysphonia is a common symptom of a:

   a. Tumor of the bronchioles.

   b. Tumor of the lung.

   c. Tumor of the larynx.

   d. None of the above

2. Nasal polyps are growths that form from distended mucous membranes and protrude into the:

   a. Sinus cavity.

   b. Throat.

   c. Nasal cavity.

   d. None of the above.

3. A pulmonary abscess is an area of contained _____ in the lung.

   a. Fluid

b. Infectious material

c. Tissue

d. None of the above

4. Histoplasmosis is a _____ disease originating in the lungs, with greatest occurrence in the Midwestern United States.

   a. Bacterial

   b. Fungal

   c. Viral

   d. None of the above

5. A pneumothorax is a collection of air or gas in the pleural cavity that can cause:

   a. A collapsed lung.

   b. Lung cancer.

   c. A bacterial infection.

   d. All of the above.

6. Infectious mononucleosis is caused by:

   a. Epstein-Barr virus.

   b. Histoplasmosis.

   c. Bacteria.

   d. None of the above.

7. Organism-specific antibiotics are used to treat:

   a. Histoplasmosis.

   b. Mononucleosis.

   c. Bacterial pneumonia.

   d. All of the above.

8. Exposure to _____ smoke may make an individual more susceptible to any respiratory condition.

   a. Primary

   b. Secondary

   c. Both a and b

   d. None of the above

9. Pneumoconiosis is caused from inhalation of:

   a. An airborne virus.

   b. Moisture droplets.

   c. Inorganic dust.

   d. All of the above.

10. Examples of occupational diseases include:

    a. Pneumonia, sinusitis, and rhinitis.

    b. Asbestosis, anthracosis, and silicosis.

    c. Flail chest, pulmonary abscess, and emphysema.

    d. None of the above.

11. Legionellosis is a more severe form of Pontiac fever, and both forms are:

    a. Contagious.

    b. Not contagious.

    c. Congenital.

    d. None of the above.

12. Barrel chest, chronic cough, and dyspnea are all symptoms of:

    a. Emphysema.

    b. Pneumonia.

    c. Hemothorax.

    d. None of the above.

13. With flail chest there are _____ fractures of three or more adjacent ribs.

    a. Single

    b. Double

    c. Both a and b

    d. Neither a nor b

14. Sinusotomy, antibiotics, and decongestants may all be treatments for:

    a. Sinusitis.

    b. Bronchitis.

    c. Allergic rhinitis.

    d. None of the above.

15. There are almost 200 different viruses that are responsible for causing:

    a. Sinusitis.

    b. Bronchitis.

    c. The common cold.

    d. None of the above.

16. In the Southwest coccidioidomycosis is caused by a fungus, *Coccidioides immitis*. This is the agent that causes the disease known as:

    a. Legionnaires' disease.

    b. Histoplasmosis.

    c. Valley fever.

    d. Asthma.

17. Currently a human vaccine exists for which of the following?

    a. H1N1 (swine flu)

    b. SARS (severe acute respiratory syndrome)

    c. Avian flu

    d. Respiratory syncytial virus pneumonia

18. Which of the following facts is(are) true about the health hazards of common molds?

    a. Mold in homes can cause symptoms of allergy.

    b. Mold exposure does *not* always present a health problem.

    c. All mold should be treated the same regarding potential health risks.

    d. All of the above are true.

19. An accumulation of pus or gas generated by microorganism activity in the pleural space can result in:

    a. Valley fever.

    b. Pneumothorax.

    c. Histoplasmosis.

    d. Tuberculosis.

20. The second most common cause of cancer death worldwide in men is:

    a. Colon and rectum cancer.

    b. Brain cancer.

    c. Skin cancer.

    d. None of the above.

21. Sputum removal management is most important in the treatment of:

    a. Flail chest.

    b. Bronchiectasis.

    c. Pleurisy.

    d. Pharyngitis

22. The sinuses are normally air filled. Where are the sinuses cavities located?

    a. Behind the nose, cheeks, and eye sockets

    b. Behind the tonsils, pharyngeal, and larynx.

    c. Behind the chin, tongue, and cheeks.

    d. Behind the eyes, eyebrows, and ears.

23. Which patient teaching methods should be employed with pulmonary tuberculosis?

    a. Consistent hand-washing techniques and respiratory precautions must be practiced.

    b. Patient and family education about sources of contagion and transmission.

    c. A nutritious diet and sanitary living conditions are important for recovery. Stress the importance of regular follow-up care.

    d. All of the above.

Scenario

A 56-year-old patient is having a nosebleed and does not know how to get it to stop. The patient has never had a previous nosebleed.

QUESTIONS:

a. How do you explain to the patient what to do?

_____

_____

_____

_____

_____

b. When should the patient seek medical attention?

_____

_____

_____

_____

_____

c. Should you stay on the phone with the patient until the bleeding stops?

_____

_____

_____

_____

_____

d. Should you ask how long the patient has been bleeding?

_____

_____

_____

_____

_____

160

Chapter **9** **Diseases and Conditions of the Respiratory System**

10 Diseases and Conditions of the Circulatory System

WORD DEFINITIONS

Define the following basic medical terms.

1. Ablation _____

2. Angina _____

3. Anticoagulant _____

4. Angioplasty _____

5. Antipyretic _____

6. Arteriosclerosis _____

7. Arteritis _____

8. Asystole _____

9. Atheroma _____

10. Atherosclerosis _____

11. Bradycardia _____

12. Bronchodilator _____

13. Carditis _____

14. Cardiomegaly _____

15. Cardiomyopathy _____

16. Cyanosis _____

17. Diastole _____

18. Embolism _____

19. Endocarditis _____

20. ESR _____

21. Gingival _____

22. Hyperlipidemia _____

23. Leukocytosis _____

24. Polyarthritis _____

25. Polycythemia _____

26. Serous _____

27. Systole _____

28. Tachycardia _____

29. Transdermal _____

30. Vegetation _____

GLOSSARY TERMS

Define the following chapter glossary terms.

1. Agglutination _____

2. Aggregation _____

3. Anaphylaxis _____

4. Angioplasty _____

5. Angiotensin-converting enzyme _____

6. Antibodies _____

7. Arrhythmias _____

8. Blood gas _____

9. Bruit _____

10. Coagulation _____

11. Collateral _____

12. Commissurotomy _____

13. Diuretics _____

14. Doppler _____

15. Dyscrasia _____

16. Gangrene _____

17. Hematocrit _____

18. Idiopathic _____

19. Opacity _____

20. Perfusion _____

21. Petechiae _____

22. Plaque _____

23. Prophylactic _____

24. Purpura _____

25. Rales _____

26. Sclerosing _____

27. Syncope _____

28. Tamponade _____

SHORT ANSWER

Answer the following questions.

1. The heart pumps how many quarts of blood throughout the body each minute?

   _____

2. Identify the first symptom of coronary artery disease.

   _____

3. List individuals having the potential to be at increased risk for coronary artery disease.

   _____

4. What is the term used to explain the new growth of blood vessels for patients with coronary artery disease (CAD)?

   _____

5. Describe the pain that is experienced by a patient experiencing angina pectoris.

   _____

6. Identify the forms of nitroglycerin that are helpful in preventing angina.

   _____

7. Cite the percentage of deaths occurring in the first hour after a myocardial infarction.

   _____

8. What measures are initiated to try to reverse cardiac arrest?

   _____

9. Name the most prevalent cardiovascular disorder in the United States.

   _____

10. List the symptoms of essential hypertension.

_____

11. Are people always aware that they have hypertension?

_____

12. Identify the cardiac test that helps in evaluating cardiac chamber size; ventricular function; and disease of the myocardium, valves, cardiac strictures, and pericardium.

_____

13. Cor pulmonale affects which side of the heart?

_____

14. Describe the skin of a person with pulmonary edema.

_____

15. Which type of growth on the cardiac valves characterizes endocarditis?

_____

16. Identify a preventive measure before dental work for people with endocarditis.

_____

17. Which valves of the heart can be affected by valvular heart disease?

_____

18. Identify the cause of rheumatic heart disease.

_____

_____

19. Name the final option for treating rheumatic heart disease.

_____

20. List the symptoms associated with mitral valve prolapse.

_____

21. How are cardiac arrhythmias diagnosed?

_____

22. Which part of the heart fails to work effectively during cardiogenic shock?

_____

_____

23. Explain the cause of cardiac tamponade.

_____

24. List the three forms of arteriosclerosis.

_____

25. Which form of arteriosclerosis is responsible for most myocardial and cerebral infarctions?

_____

26. In addition to blood clots, list forms of offending emboli that may occlude a blood vessel.

_____

27. List some of the possible causes of varicose veins.

_____

28. List some contributing factors to Raynaud's disease.

_____

29. List the components of blood.

_____

30. What causes hemolytic anemia?

_____

31. How are leukemias classified?

_____

32. Name the form of leukemia that is the most common adult leukemia and accounts for 20% of childhood leukemias.

_____

33. Identify the initial symptoms of Hodgkin's disease.

_____

34. List types of clotting disorders.

_____

FILL IN THE BLANKS

Fill in the blanks with the correct terms. A word list has been provided. Words used twice are indicated with a (2).

Word List
4, 6, abnormality, artery (2), atria, bacteria, blood pressure readings, bloody, breath, cardiac, cardiac,chest, chest, congestive heart failure (CHF), conduction, coughing, dyspnea (2), extravascular, fatigue, first, fluid, fungal, heart disease, heart valves, increased, insufficiency, interference, joints, limbs, lumen, muscle, oxygen supply, palpitations, plaque, rates, rheumatic fever, stenosis, striated muscle cells, tachycardia, thrombus, viral

1. The two upper chambers of the heart are called _____, and the two lower chambers are called _____.

2. Cardiac muscle tissue is composed of _____.

3. Myocardial infarction results from insufficient _____, as when a coronary _____ is occluded by atherosclerotic plaque, _____, or myocardial _____ spasm.

4. Cardiopulmonary resuscitation (CPR) must be initiated within _____ to _____ minutes of the _____ arrest.

5. Elevated _____ is(are) the _____ indication of hypertension.

6. Pulmonary edema causes patients to experience _____ and _____, orthopnea, _____ cardiac and respiratory _____, and often _____ frothy sputum.

7. Endocarditis is usually secondary to _____ in the bloodstream.

8. Almost one-third of all deaths in Western countries are attributed to _____.

9. Deposits of fat-containing substances called _____ on the _____ of the coronary arteries result in atherosclerosis.

10. Angioplasty is attempted to open up a constricted _____ in coronary artery disease.

11. Pulmonary edema is a condition of _____ shift into the _____ spaces of the lungs.

12. Cardiomyopathy causes the patient to experience symptoms of _____, _____, including _____, _____, _____, and occasionally _____ pain.

13. Myocarditis is frequently a(an) _____, bacterial, _____, or protozoal infection or complication of other diseases.

14. Valvular heart disease can occur in the form of _____ or _____.

15. Arrhythmias occur when there is _____ with the _____ system of the heart, resulting in a(an) _____ of the heartbeat.

16. With congestive heart failure, patients reporting unexplained _____ discomfort, shortness of _____, or swelling of _____ require prompt medical assessment.

17. _____ is the part of the heart that prevents blood from flowing backward.

18. _____ is a systemic inflammatory and autoimmune disease involving _____ and _____ tissue.

ANATOMIC STRUCTURES

Identify the structures in the following anatomic diagrams. For number 4, identify what occurs with each phase of the cardiac cycle.

1. Anterior view of the heart and great vessels

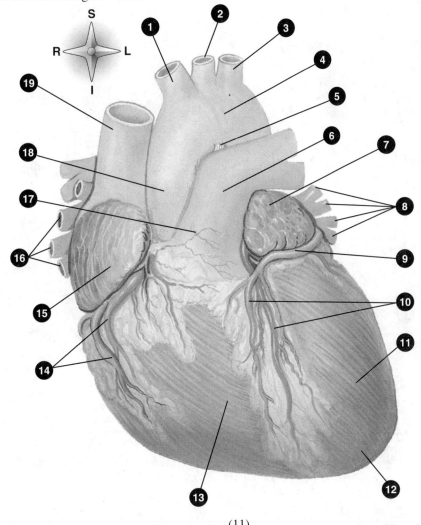

(1) _____

(2) _____

(3) _____

(4) _____

(5) _____

(6) _____

(7) _____

(8) _____

(9) _____

(10) _____

(11) _____

(12) _____

(13) _____

(14) _____

(15) _____

(16) _____

(17) _____

(18) _____

(19) _____

2. Posterior view of the heart and great vessels

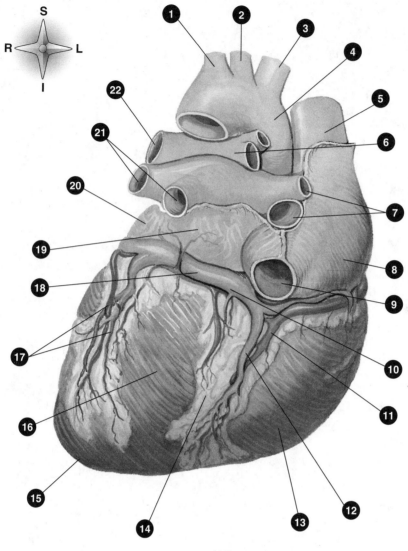

(1) _____

(2) _____

(3) _____

(4) _____

(5) _____

(6) _____

(7) _____

(8) _____

(9) _____

(10) _____

(11) _____

(12) _____

(13) _____

(14) _____

(15) _____

(16) _____

(17) _____

(18) _____

(19) _____

(20) _____

(21) _____

(22) _____

3. Circulation through the heart

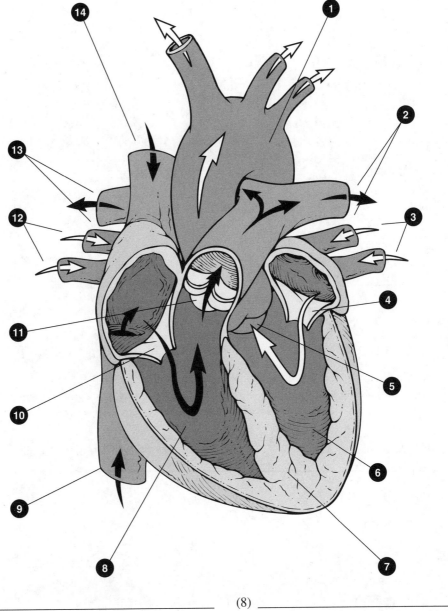

(1) _____   (8) _____

(2) _____   (9) _____

(3) _____   (10) _____

(4) _____   (11) _____

(5) _____   (12) _____

(6) _____   (13) _____

(7) _____   (14) _____

Chapter **10** **Diseases and Conditions of the Circulatory System**

4. Cardiac cycle

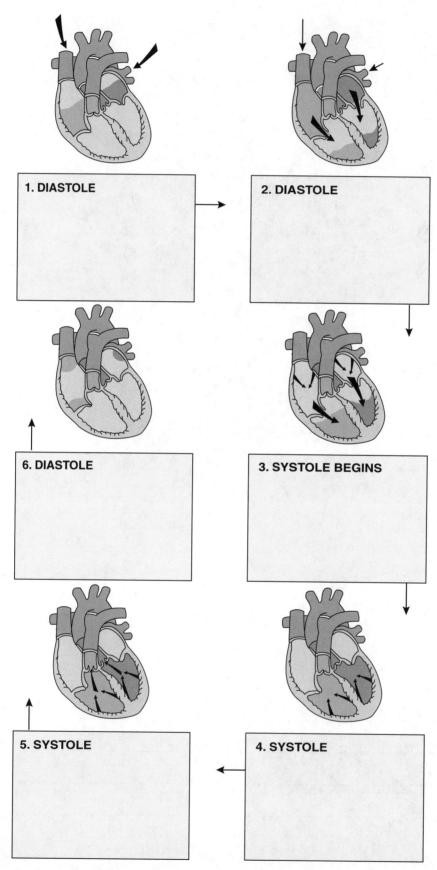

1. DIASTOLE

2. DIASTOLE

6. DIASTOLE

3. SYSTOLE BEGINS

5. SYSTOLE

4. SYSTOLE

Chapter **10**   **Diseases and Conditions of the Circulatory System**

5. Layers of the heart wall

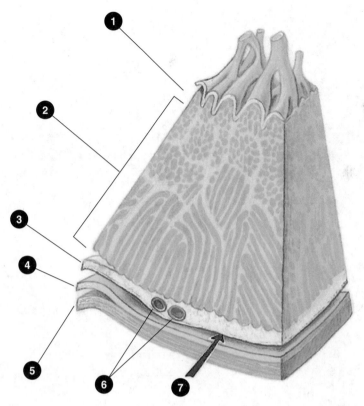

(1) _____

(2) _____

(3) _____

(4) _____

(5) _____

(6) _____

(7) _____

6. Coronary arteries

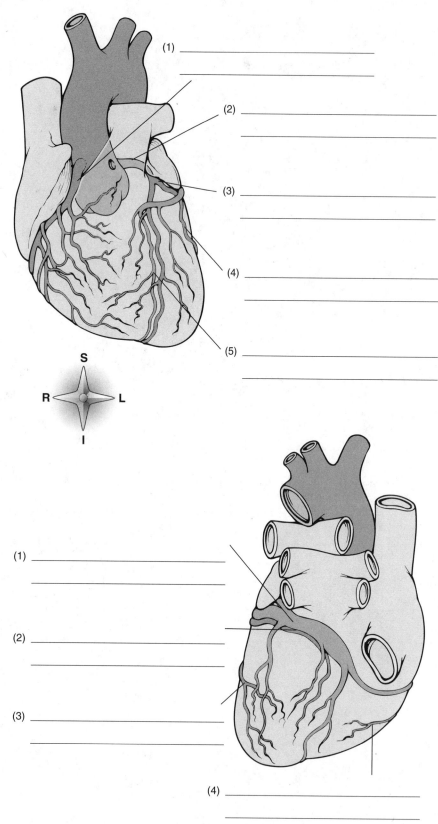

(1) _____

_____

(2) _____

_____

(3) _____

_____

(4) _____

_____

(5) _____

_____

S

R ◆ L

I

(1) _____

_____

(2) _____

_____

(3) _____

_____

(4) _____

_____

7. Conduction system of the heart

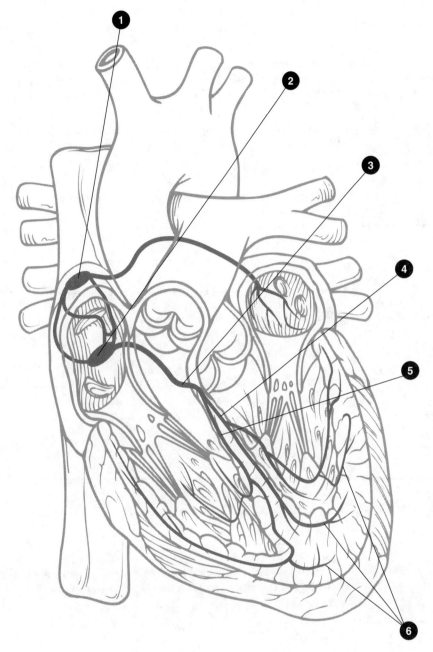

(1) _____

(2) _____

(3) _____

(4) _____

(5) _____

(6) _____

Chapter **10 Diseases and Conditions of the Circulatory System**

PATIENT SCREENING

For each of the following scenarios, explain how and why you would schedule an appointment or suggest a referral based on the patient's reported symptoms. First review the "Guidelines for Patient-Screening Exercises" found on p. iv in the Introduction.

1. A patient's wife calls stating that her husband just experienced the sudden onset of left-sided chest pain after exertion. The pain has radiated to the left arm. It was relieved when he stopped the strenuous activity and placed a nitroglycerin tablet under his tongue. She wants to know if the physician should see him. How do you handle this call?

_____

_____

_____

_____

_____

2. A patient calls saying that she is experiencing headaches, light-headedness, and dizziness. She took her blood pressure at an automatic blood pressure screening station at the pharmacy, and the reading was 168/98. How do you handle this phone call?

_____

_____

_____

_____

_____

3. The husband of a patient calls to report that his wife has started having swollen feet and ankles, weight increase, and slight shortness of breath. She has a history of congestive heart failure. How do you handle this call?

_____

_____

_____

_____

_____

4. A patient calls reporting pain and tenderness in the left leg that is becoming more severe. She has noted swelling, redness, warmth, and the development of a tender cordlike mass under the skin. How do you handle this call?

_____

_____

_____

_____

_____

_____

5. A patient calls the office and says that she is experiencing fatigue and that her skin—especially on her hands—looks pale to her. She has had a few brief episodes of shortness of breath and a "pounding heart." How do you respond to this phone call?

_____

_____

_____

_____

_____

_____

PATIENT TEACHING

For each of the following scenarios, outline the appropriate patient teaching you would perform. First review the "Guidelines for Patient-Teaching Exercises" found on p. iv in the Introduction.

1. CORONARY ARTERY DISEASE (CAD)
   A patient has recently been diagnosed with CAD. She has returned to the office for additional patient teaching concerning this condition. The office has printed material outlining emergency medical intervention in the event of chest pain and the prevention and control of the disorder. The physician asks that you provide this material to the patient and review it with her. How do you approach this patient-teaching opportunity?

_____

_____

_____

_____

2. HYPERTENSION

A patient diagnosed with hypertension is in the office for a blood pressure recheck. He makes the statement that, because his blood pressure is much better today, he can stop taking the medication. The physician asks that you reinforce his instructions that the medication still needs to be taken on a regular basis. The office has printed material available to give to hypertensive patients. How do you approach this patient-teaching opportunity?

_____

_____

_____

_____

3. CONGESTIVE HEART FAILURE (CHF)

A patient is experiencing recurring CHF. The physician asks you to reinforce his instructions to the patient and family regarding treatment of the condition. How do you approach this patient-teaching opportunity?

_____

_____

_____

_____

4. ATHEROSCLEROSIS

A diagnosis of atherosclerosis has been confirmed. The physician requests your assistance in reinforcing her recommendations to the patient. The office has printed materials regarding this condition, and you are instructed to review these with the patient. How do you approach this patient-teaching opportunity?

_____

_____

_____

_____

5. RAYNAUD'S PHENOMENON

It is a very cold day, and the patient has just seen the physician after a severe attack of her condition. Even though the physician has previously advised her about the importance of avoiding situations in which she is exposed to severe cold, she continues to go outside without gloves and head covering. The physician asks you to provide the patient with printed information concerning her condition and reinforce the fact that exposure to severe cold will cause severe pain. How do you approach this patient-teaching opportunity?

_____

_____

_____

_____

6. CORORNARY ARTERY DISEASE
   Describe three different coronary artery preventative measures to help patients with this diagnosis.

   _____

   _____

   _____

   _____

7. Explain patient screening for patients experiencing symptoms of angina for the first time.

   _____

   _____

   _____

   _____

8. Identify the patient teaching to a patient with myocarditis.

   _____

   _____

   _____

   _____

PHARMACOLOGY QUESTIONS

Circle the letter of the choice that best completes the statement or answers the question.

1. Angina pectoris is commonly treated with sublingual nitroglycerin tablets. Which of the following is correct concerning the use of nitroglycerin?

   a. May be repeated every five minutes to relieve angina if no relief.

   b. Sublingual tablets are not kept in the original glass container.

   c. Tablets should not be kept in the refrigerator after opening.

   d. Sublingual tablets are not explosive and should be handled carefully.

2. Cardiac arrest is the sudden unexpected cessation of the heart. Which of the following interventions would be expected to be taken after cardiac arrest?

   a. Lidocaine injection

   b. CPR

   c. Sublingual beta-adrenergic drugs

   d. Both A and b

3. Which of the following medications is not commonly used to treat hypertension?

 a. Candesartan (Atacand)

 b. Glyburide (DiaBeta)

 c. Atenolol (Tenormin)

 d. Furosemide (Lasix)

4. Which of the following drugs should be avoided in a patient with hypertension?

 a. Hydrochlorothiazide

 b. Lisinopril (Zestril)

 c. Pseudoephedrine (Sudafed)

 d. Verapamil (Calan)

5. Congestive heart failure (CHF) is frequently treated with which of the following medications?

 a. Vasodilators

 b. Beta blockers

 c. Digoxin

 d. All of the above

6. The use of which of the following medicines is discouraged when a patient is taking nitrate-based vasodilators?

 a. Hydrochlorothiazide

 b. Beta blockers

 c. Sildenafil (Viagra)

 d. Calcium channel blockers

7. Which of the following medications may be used in the treatment of cardiomyopathy?

 a. Digoxin (Lanoxin)

 b. Warfarin (Coumadin)

 c. Metformin (Glucophage)

 d. Both a and b

8. Medications used to treat endocarditis would most often include (best answer):

 a. Antiinflammatories.

 b. Antibiotics.

 c. Antipyretics.

 d. Antifungals.

9. Which of the following drugs would be best at preventing thrombi?

 a. Digoxin (Lanoxin)

 b. Dicyclomine (Bentyl)

 c. Dexamethasone (Decadron)

 d. Warfarin (Coumadin)

178

10. Which of the following treatments would not be acceptable for the treatment of shock?

    a. Elevating the legs

    b. Replacing IV fluids

    c. Applying ice packs

    d. Maintaining proper ventilation

11. Which of the following is not a drug used to treat elevated cholesterol levels?

    a. Simvastatin (Zocor)

    b. Ezetimibe (Zetia)

    c. Niacin

    d. Methylprednisolone (Medrol)

12. Which of the following statements is true?

    a. Heparin can be given orally or intravenously.

    b. Warfarin has a faster onset of action.

    c. Heparin is given by injection only.

    d. Warfarin comes in only one tablet strength.

13. Which of the following medications is(are) frequently used in the treatment of anemia?

    a. Iron

    b. Folic acid

    c. Vitamin B_{12} (cyanocobalamin)

    d. All of the above

14. What part of the heart prevents the blood from flowing backward?

ESSAY QUESTION

Write a response to the following question or statement. Use a separate sheet of paper if more space is needed.

1. Describe the laboratory tests that are used to confirm a diagnosis of acute lymphocytic leukemia (ALL).

_____

_____

_____

_____

_____

_____

_____

_____

2. Describe the three changes in enzyme levels that indicate the death of cardias tissue.

_____

_____

_____

_____

_____

_____

_____

3. Compare the cause of cor pulmonale to the cause of pulmonary edema.

_____

_____

_____

_____

_____

_____

_____

_____

CERTIFICATION EXAMINATION REVIEW

Circle the letter of the choice that best completes the statement or answers the question.

1. A person who complains of experiencing chest pain with exertion is having:

    a. Angina pectoris.

    b. A myocardial infarction.

    c. Shortness of breath.

    d. None of the above.

2. Pericarditis is an inflammation of the:

    a. Myocardium.

    b. Endocardium.

    c. Sac enclosing the heart.

    d. None of the above.

3. Raynaud's disease is a vasospastic disease that affects the:

   a. Heart.

   b. Legs and arms.

   c. Hands, fingers, and feet.

   d. None of the above.

4. The diagnosis of anemia indicates that the patient is experiencing a reduction in:

   a. Red blood cells or hemoglobin.

   b. Platelets.

   c. Lymphatic tissue.

   d. None of the above.

5. In which ethnic group is sickle cell anemia most prominently diagnosed?

   a. African American.

   b. Native American.

   c. Asian.

   d. None of the above.

6. The lymphatic tissue in Hodgkin's disease patients contains:

   a. Sickle cells.

   b. Monocytes.

   c. Reed-Sternberg cells.

   d. None of the above.

7. Rheumatic heart disease may cause problems with the:

   a. Myocardium.

   b. Valves.

   c. Atria.

   d. None of the above.

8. Left-sided crushing-type chest pain, irregular heartbeat, dyspnea, excessive sweating, nausea, anxiety, and denial are all symptoms of:

   a. Mitral stenosis.

   b. Angina pectoris.

   c. Myocardial infarction.

   d. All of the above.

9. Electrocution, myocardial infarction, and drug overdose may cause:

   a. Hypertension.

   b. Cardiac arrest.

   c. Cardiomyopathy.

   d. None of the above.

10. People with mitral valve prolapse are sometimes:

   a. Asymptomatic.

   b. Anxious.

   c. Experiencing heart palpitations.

   d. All of the above.

11. Primary or essential hypertension:

   a. Is related to lifestyle habits.

   b. Is genetic.

   c. Has an unknown etiology.

   d. None of the above.

12. Ischemia causes:

   a. Death to tissue.

   b. Swelling of tissue.

   c. Blood disorders.

   d. None of the above.

13. Blood transfusion incompatibility reactions are:

   a. Potentially life threatening.

   b. Always fatal.

   c. A common problem.

   d. None of the above.

14. Lymphedema causes swelling of:

   a. The heart.

   b. An extremity.

   c. Heart valves.

   d. None of the above.

15. Cardiac arrhythmias are the result of:

   a. Smoking.

   b. Fat deposits.

   c. Interference with the conduction system of the heart.

   d. None of the above.

16. Patients with coronary artery disease, while still very preliminary to stimulate new growth of blood vessels, how is deoxyribonucleic acid (DNA) administered?

   a. Inserted with a stent

   b. Taken orally

   c. Injection directly into cardiac muscle

   d. Inserted with a balloon

182

17. While the cause of essential hypertension is unknown, there are many factors thought to contribute to the condition. What is considered to be the major factor in hypertension?

    a. Poor dietary habits

    b. Stress

    c. Age

    d. Smoking

Scenario

Scenario will require students to use critical thinking skills to determine the various possible answers. Some research may be necessary to include an evidence-based answer.

    A family rushed their mother to the emergency room with chest pain, shortness of breath, and the feeling of a heart attack. The emergency room ran many tests and admitted the mother with a diagnosis of Broken Heart Syndrome. The family member has never heard of that diagnosis and needs more clarification. How would you help the family understand the following questions?

a. What is Broken Heart Syndrome?

_____

_____

_____

_____

b. Why does this happen?

_____

_____

_____

_____

c. What causes the symptoms?

_____

_____

_____

_____

d. What kind of incident?

_____

_____

_____

_____

e. How are they able to tell it isn't a heart attack?

_____

_____

_____

_____

f. What can be done for my mother now?

_____

_____

_____

_____

g. Is my mother going to get better?

_____

_____

_____

_____

h. What can I do for my mother?

_____

_____

_____

_____

11 Diseases and Conditions of the Urinary System

WORD DEFINITIONS

Define the following basic medical terms.

1. ARF _____

2. Anorexia _____

3. BUN _____

4. Calculi _____

5. Casts _____

6. Extracellular _____

7. Flank _____

8. Intrarenal _____

9. IVP _____

10. Lethargic _____

11. Micturition _____

12. Nephrolithotomy _____

13. Neuropathies _____

14. Oliguria _____

15. Pitting edema _____

16. Proteinuria _____

17. Renin _____

18. Retroperitoneally _____

19. Spontaneously _____

20. Urgency _____

21. Urination _____

22. Catheterization _____

23. Cystoscopy _____

24. Glomerulonephritis _____

25. Glomerulosclerosis _____

26. Hemodialysis _____

27. Hydronephrosis _____

28. Immunosuppressive _____

29. Lithotripsy _____

30. Nephrectomy _____

31. Nephrotoxic _____

32. Peritoneal dialysis _____

33. Pyelonephritis _____

GLOSSARY TERMS

Define the following chapter glossary terms.

1. Azotemia _____

2. BUN _____

3. Calculi _____

4. Clean-catch urine specimen _____

5. Dialysis _____

6. Erythrocyte sedimentation rate (ESR) _____

7. Fibrotic _____

8. Glomerulosclerosis _____

9. Glomeruli _____

10. Hematuria _____

11. Hypoalbuminemia _____

12. Idiopathic _____

13. Intravenous pyelograms _____

14. Intravenous urogram _____

15. Malaise _____

16. Metabolic acidosis   _____

17. Nephrons   _____

18. Pyelonephritis   _____

19. Renal calculi   _____

20. Uremia   _____

SHORT ANSWER

Answer the following questions.

1. Why does chronic glomerulonephritis lead to renal failure?

   _____

2. What diagnostic test is often ordered to evaluate the function of the urinary system?

   _____

3. What usually precedes acute glomerulonephritis?

   _____

4. Name the procedure used to examine the urinary tract.

   _____

5. What causes the symptoms of renal calculi to vary?

   _____

6. What is the most common type of kidney disease?

   _____

7. List causes of neurogenic bladder.

   _____

8. Describe hematuria.

   _____

9. List the functions of the urinary system.

   _____

10. Pressure from urine that cannot flow past an obstruction in the urinary tract causes what condition that affects the kidney?

   _____

11. List types of nephrotoxic agents that commonly cause renal damage.

_____

_____

12. Name the treatment of choice for renal cell carcinoma.

_____

13. Define nephrotic syndrome.

_____

14. Glomerulosclerosis results from which disease?

_____

15. List usual causes of cystitis and urethritis.

_____

_____

16. In relation to the urinary system, list the occasions when catheterization may be indicated.

_____

_____

17. Define pyuria.

_____

18. List the symptoms of acute glomerulonephritis.

_____

19. List factors that may lead to stress incontinence (enuresis).

_____

_____

20. Identify the cause of bladder cancer.

_____

21. Describe the sequence of events when a patient has acute renal failure.

_____

_____

22. When a patient has hydronephrosis, after what length of time will a kidney fail to function if an obstruction is not resolved?

_____

23. Explain the usual treatment of renal calculi.

_____

24. Identify the cause of polycystic kidney disease.

_____

25. Describe the appearance of a polycystic kidney.

_____

_____

26. Describe the composition of a nephron.

_____

27. Describe the responsibility of the neurons.

_____

28. Discuss the location of the kidneys.

_____

29. Name the three regions of each kidney.

_____

30. Trace the flow of blood through the kidneys in the formation of urine.

_____

31. Trace the flow of urine as it leaves the kidneys.

_____

32. What is the nephrons function in the kidney?

_____

33. Explain how extracorporeal shock wave lithrotripsy (ESWL) is beneficial in renal calculi.

_____

34. Explain the way infectious cystitis and urethritis can be transmitted.

_____

35. Each kidney is composed of about 1 million microstructures called nephrons. What are the nephrons function in the kidney?

_____

36. What are the three main goals in the treatment of bladder cancer?

_____

FILL IN THE BLANKS

Fill in the blanks with the correct terms. A word list has been provided. Words used twice are indicated with a (2).

Word List

acute glomerulonephritis, antibiotics, bladder, blood tests, bloody urine, calcium, cephalosporin, decreased urinary output, drowsiness, excreting urine, failure, filtration, gastrointestinal disturbances, glomerular, glucose, headache, hypertension, individualized, inflammatory, kidneys (2), nausea, nephron, normalcy, oliguria, penicillin, pressure, producing, protein losing, reabsorption, secretion, storing, ureters, urethra, uric acid, urinalysis, urinary bladder, urinary tract infections (UTIs)

1. With renal cell carcinoma, the malignancy can begin in the _____ or be secondary to carcinoma elsewhere in the body.

2. The urinary system is responsible for _____, _____, and _____.

3. The functional unit of the kidney is the _____.

4. The three functional processes of the kidney in the manufacture of urine are _____, _____, and _____.

5. Urine is stored in the _____.

6. Function of the urinary system is evaluated by _____ and _____.

7. Four symptoms of urinary disease are _____, _____ _____, _____, and _____.

8. _____ is an inflammation and swelling of the glomeruli.

9. The major structures of the urinary system consist of _____ _____, two _____, the _____ _____, and the _____.

10. Nephrotic syndrome encompasses a group of symptoms referred to as _____ kidney.

11. Initial symptoms of acute renal failure include _____, _____, _____, and other alterations in the level of consciousness.

12. The treatment of choice for pyelonephritis consists of intravenous or oral _____, usually _____ or _____, given for a full 7 to 10 days.

13. Kidney stones form when there is an excessive amount of _____ or _____ in the blood.

14. Patients with diabetes vary in their susceptibility to renal _____; thus the treatment plan for diabetic glomerulosclerosis is _____ for each person.

15. The treatment for neurogenic bladder is directed toward prevention of _____ and attempts to restore some _____ in function.

16. Immune mechanisms are suspected to be a major cause of CGN; antigen-antibody complexes lodge in the glomerular capsular membrane, triggering an _____ response and _____ injury.

17. Make patients with diabetes aware of the importance of maintaining blood _____ at appropriate levels. They also should be advised about the importance of monitoring their blood _____ and keeping it at acceptable levels.

190

ANATOMIC STRUCTURES

Identify the structures in the following anatomic diagrams. For number 4, identify the three phases of urine formation.

1. The urinary system

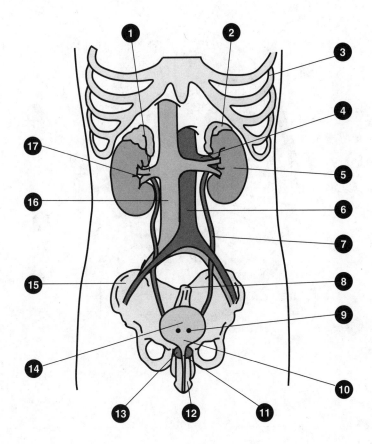

(1) _____   (10) _____

(2) _____   (11) _____

(3) _____   (12) _____

(4) _____   (13) _____

(5) _____   (14) _____

(6) _____   (15) _____

(7) _____   (16) _____

(8) _____   (17) _____

(9) _____

2. Internal structure of the kidney

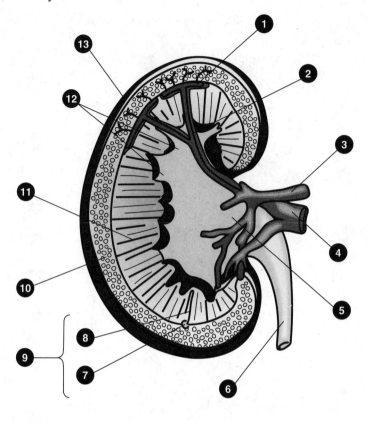

(1) _____   (8) _____

(2) _____   (9) _____

(3) _____   (10) _____

(4) _____   (11) _____

(5) _____   (12) _____

(6) _____   (13) _____

(7) _____

3. The nephron

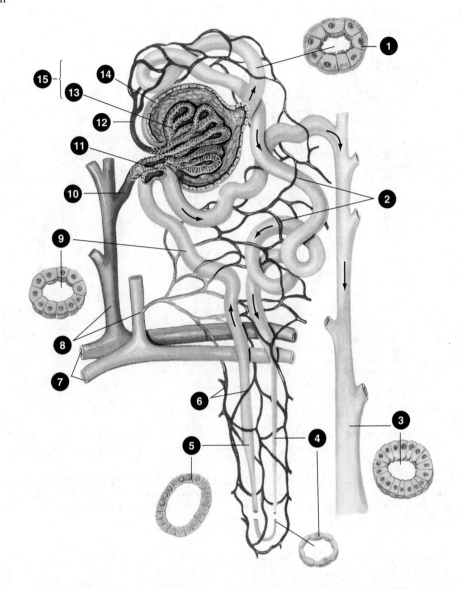

(1) _____

(2) _____

(3) _____

(4) _____

(5) _____

(6) _____

(7) _____

(8) _____

(9) _____

(10) _____

(11) _____

(12) _____

(13) _____

(14) _____

(15) _____

4. Formation of urine

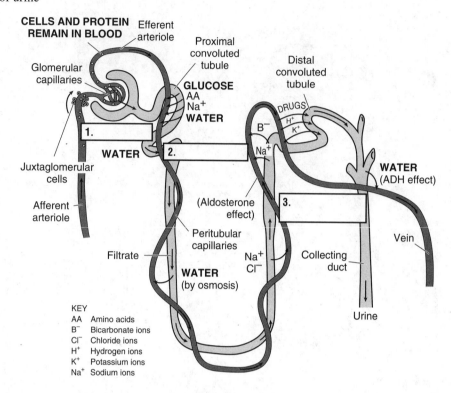

CELLS AND PROTEIN
REMAIN IN BLOOD   Efferent
                     arteriole
                                  Proximal
                                  convoluted
                                  tubule   Distal
Glomerular   convoluted
capillaries   GLUCOSE   tubule
                             AA
                             Na⁺   DRUGS
                             WATER   H⁺
                                           B⁻   K⁺
            1.   Na⁺
                     WATER   2.
                                                                WATER
Juxtaglomerular   (ADH effect)
cells

Afferent   (Aldosterone   3.
arteriole   effect)

                     Peritubular   Vein
                     capillaries
         Filtrate   Na⁺   Collecting
                                            Cl⁻   duct
                     WATER
                     (by osmosis)
                                                            Urine
         KEY
         AA   Amino acids
         B⁻   Bicarbonate ions
         Cl⁻ Chloride ions
         H⁺   Hydrogen ions
         K⁺   Potassium ions
         Na⁺ Sodium ions

PATIENT SCREENING

For each of the following scenarios, explain how and why you would schedule an appointment or suggest a referral based on the patient's reported symptoms. First review the "Guidelines for Patient-Screening Exercises" found on p. iv in the Introduction.

1. A mother calls to report that her daughter has experienced a sudden onset of extremely bloody urine. The urine is dark and is described as being coffee colored. The child had a streptococcal infection 1 to 2 weeks ago. She also is complaining of a headache, has a loss of appetite, and has a low-grade fever. Flank or back pain is an additional complaint of the child. How do you handle this call?

_____

_____

_____

_____

2. A patient reports that she has experienced rapid onset of fever, chills, nausea and vomiting, and flank (lumbar) pain. She had a UTI with urinary frequency and urgency last week. The patient reports a foul odor to the urine with possible blood and pus. There is tenderness in the suprapubic region. How do you handle this call?

_____

_____

_____

_____

3. A patient calls advising that he has experienced sudden severe pain in the flank area and urinary urgency. He also complains of nausea and vomiting, blood in the urine, fever, chills, and abdominal distention. How do you respond to this phone call?

_____

_____

_____

_____

4. A female patient calls the office complaining of urinary urgency, frequency, and even incontinence. In addition, she says that she has pain in the pelvic region and low back, bladder spasms, fever and chills, and a burning sensation with urination. Her urine is dark yellow. How do you respond to this phone call?

_____

_____

_____

_____

5. A female patient advises that she is experiencing leakage of urine on coughing, sneezing, laughing, lifting, or running without prior urgency. She is unable to control the leakage during physical exertion. How do you handle this call?

_____

_____

_____

_____

PATIENT TEACHING

For each of the following scenarios, outline the appropriate patient teaching you would perform. First review the "Guidelines for Patient-Teaching Exercises" found on p. iv in the Introduction.

1. ACUTE GLOMERULONEPHRITIS
   A patient has recently been diagnosed with acute glomerulonephritis. Antibiotics have been prescribed. The physician has printed instructions for patients with this condition. You are asked to give the patient and family the printed information and review it with them. How do you approach this patient-teaching opportunity?

_____

_____

_____

_____

2. PYELONEPHRITIS

A female patient has a recurring occurrence of pyelonephritis. The physician has asked you to provide and review this material with her. How do you approach this patient-teaching opportunity?

_____

_____

_____

_____

3. RENAL CALCULI

A patient complains of sudden onset of severe flank pain accompanied by pelvic pressure. Radiographs indicate the presence of renal calculi. The physician asks you to give the patient printed information concerning renal calculi therapy. How do you approach this patient-teaching opportunity?

_____

_____

_____

_____

4. DIABETIC NEPHROPATHY

A patient has recently been diagnosed with diabetic neuropathy. He is somewhat confused about this complication of his diabetes. The physician has written information for this type of disorder. You are instructed to give him the printed information and review its contents with him. How do you approach this patient-teaching opportunity?

_____

_____

_____

_____

5. STRESS INCONTINENCE

A female patient has been experiencing stress incontinence. The physician has printed instructions to help patients deal with this condition. The physician asks that you give the instructions to the patient and review them with her. How do you approach this patient-teaching opportunity?

_____

_____

_____

_____

6. DIABETES

A patient has recently been diagnosed with diabetes and has never heard of the methods to monitor diabetes. While multiple reading materials can be distributed, it is important you explain the process and task of monitoring diabetes regularly. How will you advise the importance of maintaining blood levels and pressure?

_____

_____

_____

_____

7. STRESS INCONTINENCE

A female patient has been experiencing stress incontinence. The physician has printed instructions to help patients deal with this condition. The physician asks that you give the instructions to the patient and review them with her. How do you approach this patient-teaching opportunity?

_____

_____

_____

_____

8. CYSTITIS AND URETHRITIS

Explain to a patient the way infectious cystitis and urethritis can be transmitted and how to prevent these infections.

_____

_____

_____

_____

PHARMACOLOGY QUESTIONS

Circle the letter of the choice that best completes the statement or answers the question.

1. Which of the following medications may cause nephrotoxicity?

   a. Cyclosporine (Neoral)

   b. Amphotericin B

   c. Acetaminophen (Tylenol)

   d. All of the above

2. Treatment of UTIs may include all of the following therapies except:

   a. Sulfamethoxazole/trimethoprim (Bactrim).

   b. Amoxicillin (Amoxil).

   c. Reduced fluid intake.

   d. Phenazopyridine (Pyridium).

3. Urinary incontinence caused by muscle spasms of the bladder may be treated with:

   a. Cyclobenzaprine (Flexeril).

   b. Oxybutynin (Ditropan).

   c. Tolterodine (Detrol).

   d. Both b and c.

ESSAY QUESTION

Write a response to the following question or statement. Use a separate sheet of paper if more space is needed.

1. Compare hemodialysis and peritoneal dialysis.

_____

_____

_____

_____

_____

_____

_____

_____

_____

_____

_____

_____

_____

_____

2. Because there is no total cure for CRF, preventing complications and providing supportive care are important. What are the causative factors to promptly treat ARF?

_____

_____

_____

_____

_____

3. What does ESWL stand for? Explain how it is beneficial in renal calculi.

_____

_____

_____

_____

_____

4. Describe the treatment and prognosis for patients with hydronephrosis.

_____

_____

_____

_____

_____

5. Describe symptoms and signs of kidney stones.

_____

_____

_____

_____

6. Explain two treatment options used for ESRD.

_____

_____

_____

_____

CERTIFICATION EXAMINATION REVIEW

Circle the letter of the choice that best completes the statement or answers the question.

1. Obstructive diseases of the kidney may be caused by:

   a. Metabolic disorders.

   b. Congenital or structural defects.

   c. Immunologic disorders.

   d. Excessive fluid intake.

2. The most common type of renal disease is:

   a. Acute renal failure.

   b. Nephrosis.

   c. Pyelonephritis.

   d. Hydronephrosis.

3. Symptoms of cystitis include:

   a. Urinary urgency, frequency, and incontinence.

   b. Pelvic pain.

   c. Burning with urination.

   d. All of the above.

4. Group A beta-hemolytic streptococcus may precede:

   a. Hydronephrosis.

   b. Acute renal failure.

   c. Acute glomerulonephritis.

   d. Renal calculi.

5. Lithotripsy, relief of pain, surgical intervention, increased fluid intake, and diuretics are all ways of treating:

   a. Hydronephrosis.

   b. Renal calculi.

   c. Glomerulonephritis.

   d. All of the above.

6. An ascending bacterial invasion of the urinary tract can cause:

   a. Renal calculi.

   b. Hydronephrosis.

   c. Cystitis and urethritis.

   d. All of the above.

7. Chronic glomerulonephritis is:

   a. Slowly progressive and infectious.

   b. Slowly progressive and noninfectious.

   c. Not progressive.

   d. Rapidly progressive.

8. Enuresis is caused from a weakening of:

   a. The pelvic floor muscles.

   b. The urethral structure.

   c. Both a and b.

   d. Renal calculi.

9. Solvents, heavy metals, antibiotics, pesticides, and mushrooms are known to:

   a. Cause renal damage.

   b. Cause cystitis.

   c. Cause pyelonephritis.

   d. Cause renal calculi.

10. Smoking, obesity, and prolonged exposure to chemicals such as asbestos and cadmium may cause:

    a. Polycystic kidney disease.

    b. Renal cell carcinoma.

    c. Glomerulonephritis.

    d. Renal calculi.

11. Pus in the urine is called:

    a. Azotemia.

    b. Pyuria.

    c. Cystitis.

    d. Hematuria.

12. Hematuria is:

    a. Bacteria in the urine.

    b. Blood in the urine.

    c. Fat in the urine.

    d. Pus in the urine.

13. Azotemia is:

    a. A drug that promotes urine output.

    b. Excess urea in the blood.

    c. Excess urea in the urine.

    d. Excess fat in the urine.

14. A clinical emergency that involves the renal system is:

    a. Cystitis.

    b. Hematuria.

    c. Acute renal failure.

    d. Pyelonephritis.

Scenario

Parents of 5 1/2-year-old twins, a girl and a boy, bring the twins in for a check-up, but the real reason that prompted the visit is bedwetting. The parents have normal concerns of usually healthy twins. Both children are examined, with usual testing to rule out any infections. The physician requests to speak to the parent without the children present. The physician asks what, if anything, has been attempted to help prevent the enuresis. The parents stated waking up both children, restricting fluid, routine bed times, some form of small punishment (withholding a special toy), awards stickers, and comparison discussions with other siblings and cousins. Parents stated they are becoming extremely frustrated at this time and would appreciate any solution so the twins do not miss out on friend sleepover events. The physician is straightforward and informs the parents the cause of enuresis is deep sleep and children are not aware of the urge to urinate, then attempts to help stop bedwetting.

QUESTION:

What does the doctor offer to the parents as a treatment for this problem? Research on the internet for successful known treatments.

12 Diseases and Conditions of the Reproductive System

WORD DEFINITIONS

Define the following basic medical terms.

1. Amenorrhea _____

2. Anomaly _____

3. Axillary _____

4. Cervicitis _____

5. Cystitis _____

6. Cystoscopy _____

7. Degenerative _____

8. Endometrial _____

9. Lymphadenectomy _____

10. Melena _____

11. Nocturia _____

12. Noninvasive _____

13. Proctoscopy _____

14. Prostatitis _____

15. Septicemia _____

16. Urethritis _____

GLOSSARY TERMS

Define the following chapter glossary terms.

1. Abruptio placentae _____

2. Amniotic fluid _____

3. Asymptomatic _____

4. Colporrhaphy   _____

5. Endometrium   _____

6. Laparoscopy   _____

7. Neoplasm   _____

8. Nulliparous   _____

9. Pathologist   _____

10. *Peau d'orange*   _____

11. Pelvic inflammatory disease _____

12. Peritonitis   _____

13. Prostate-specific antigen _____

14. Serology, serologic   _____

15. Zygote   _____

SHORT ANSWER

Answer the following questions.

1. Name the male reproductive organs that produce sperm.

   _____

2. Identify the drug of choice to treat syphilis.

   _____

3. List the signs and symptoms of preeclampsia in pregnancy.

   _____

   _____

4. Identify the first sign of testicular cancer.

   _____

5. What is dysmenorrhea?

   _____

6. Name the term for pain that occurs at ovulation.

   _____

7. Name the sexually transmitted disease that is referred to as the *silent STD*.

_____

8. Identify the treatment for condylomata.

_____

9. What happens during placenta previa?

_____

10. Identify the second leading cause of cancer deaths among women.

_____

11. What is the best prevention of epididymitis?

_____

12. Identify the treatment for testicular torsion.

_____

13. List complications of benign prostatic hypertrophy.

_____

14. Testicular cancer is most common in men of what age?

_____

15. Cite causes of secondary dysmenorrhea.

_____

16. What is a leiomyoma?

_____

17. What is included in the diagnostic evaluation for prostate cancer?

_____

_____

18. Is dyspareunia more common in men or women?

_____

19. Identify the main goals of treatment for genital herpes.

_____

20. By what route is genital herpes transmitted?

_____

21. What, other than physical problems, can contribute to impotence?

_____

22. With regular unprotected intercourse for 1 year, what percentage of couples is able to conceive?

_____

23. What is the age range during which most women are diagnosed with ovarian cancer?

_____

24. Identify the time during pregnancy that most women experience morning sickness.

_____

25. With ectopic pregnancy, where does the fertilized ovum usually implant?

_____

26. List the characteristics of eclampsia.

_____

27. What is the difference between a complete and incomplete hydatidiform mole?

_____

28. Is cystic disease of the breast considered a benign or cancerous condition?

_____

FILL IN THE BLANKS

Fill in the blanks with the correct terms. A word list has been provided.

Word List

45, 55, acute, anterior, bacterial, breasts, burn, cheeks, cystocele, downward, ductus deferens, ejaculatory, endometrial, eye sockets, injury, itch, Kegel, genitourinary, lower, nose, prostate, protozoal, reproduction, staphylococcal, strains, streptococcal, systemic, tumors, United States, uterine, uterus, viral, women

1. Sperm is transported from the testes through the series of ducts beginning with the epididymis, the _____, and the _____ ducts.

2. The _____ are accessory organs of _____ and are two milk-producing glands.

3. Sexually transmitted disease (STD) rates in the _____ are among the highest in the world and growing.

4. Trichomoniasis is a(an) _____ infection of the lower _____ tract.

5. Genital warts are usually painless, but they may _____ or _____.

6. The most common diseases of the male reproductive system are those affecting the _____ gland.

7. _____ or _____ infection or _____ causes inflammation of the testes.

8. In endometriosis functioning _____ tissue grows outside of the _____ cavity.

9. Leiomyomas are the most common _____ of the female reproductive system.

10. Toxic shock syndrome is an acute _____ infection with toxin producing _____ of *Staphylococcus aureus*.

11. Many _____ experience the onset of menopause between the ages of _____ and _____.

12. Prolapse of the uterus is a _____ displacement of the uterus _____ from its normal location in the pelvis.

13. A _____ is a downward displacement of the urinary bladder into the _____ wall of the vagina.

14. Exercises to strengthen the pelvic floor muscles are called _____ exercises.

15. Mastitis is frequently caused by a(an) _____ infection.

16. Sinus cavities are normally air filled and located behind the _____, _____, and _____.

ANATOMIC STRUCTURES

Identify the structures in the following anatomic diagrams.

1. Normal male reproductive system

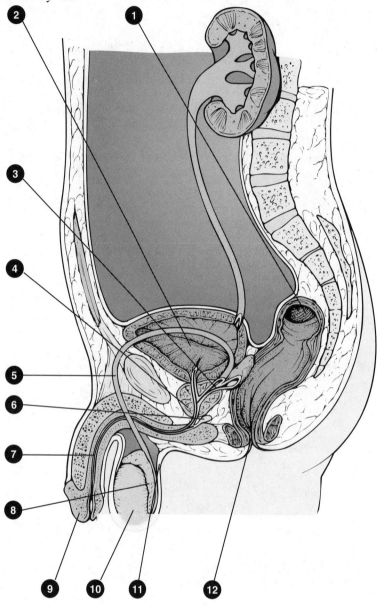

(1) _____

(2) _____

(3) _____

(4) _____

(5) _____

(6) _____

(7) _____

(8) _____

(9) _____

(10) _____

(11) _____

(12) _____

2. Normal female reproductive system

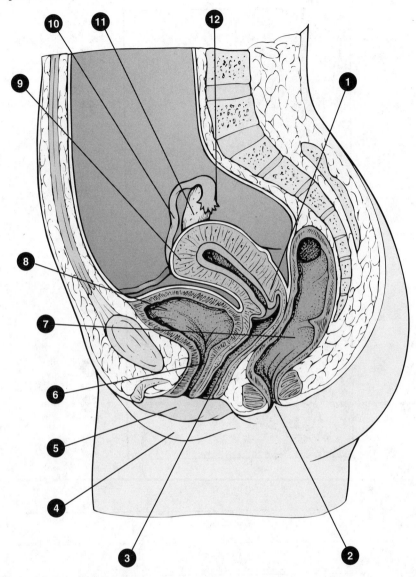

(1) _____   (7) _____

(2) _____   (8) _____

(3) _____   (9) _____

(4) _____   (10) _____

(5) _____   (11) _____

(6) _____   (12) _____

Chapter **12** **Diseases and Conditions of the Reproductive System**

3. Normal female breast

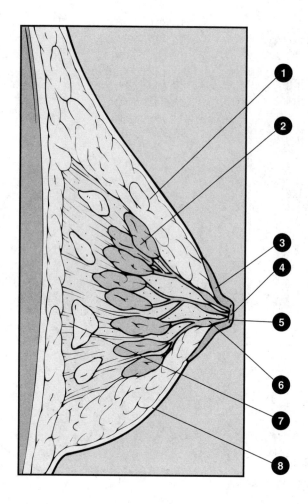

(1) _____

(2) _____

(3) _____

(4) _____

(5) _____

(6) _____

(7) _____

(8) _____

PATIENT SCREENING

For each of the following scenarios, explain how and why you would schedule an appointment or suggest a referral based on the patient's reported symptoms. First review the "Guidelines for Patient-Screening Exercises" found on p. iv in the Introduction.

1. A female patient calls to request an appointment saying that she is experiencing painful urination and severe itching in the perineal region. How do you respond to her call?

_____

_____

_____

2. A 60-year-old male patient calls the office advising that he is experiencing urinary frequency, including nocturia. How do you handle this call?

_____

_____

_____

3. A female patient calls advising that she is experiencing fever; chills; a foul-smelling vaginal discharge; backache; and a painful, tender abdomen. How do you handle this call?

_____

_____

_____

4. A female patient's husband calls the office saying that his wife is 2 months pregnant and has developed vaginal bleeding and pelvic pain from cramping. How do you handle this call?

_____

_____

_____

5. A female patient calls to request an appointment, stating that she has been experiencing an uncomfortable feeling in her breasts. She found a lump this morning in her right breast. How do you handle this call?

_____

_____

_____

PATIENT TEACHING

For each of the following scenarios, outline the appropriate patient teaching you would perform. First review the "Guidelines for Patient-Teaching Exercises" found on p. iv in the Introduction.

1. SYPHILIS

   A patient has been diagnosed with syphilis. The practice has printed instructions for patients diagnosed with this condition. The physician has instructed you to give the patient the printed information and review it with her. How do you approach this patient-teaching opportunity?

   _____

   _____

   _____

   _____

   _____

   _____

2. ORCHITIS

   A young male patient has just been diagnosed with orchitis. The physician asks you to give him the printed information concerning this condition. How do you approach this patient-teaching opportunity?

   _____

   _____

   _____

   _____

   _____

   _____

3. PREMENSTRUAL SYNDROME (PMS)

   A female patient complains of typical premenstrual syndrome symptoms. The office has printed information for patient teaching about this condition. The physician asks you to give the information sheets to the patient and review them with her. How do you approach this patient-teaching opportunity?

   _____

   _____

   _____

   _____

   _____

   _____

4. ENDOMETRIOSIS

A young female patient has been complaining of intolerable menstrual cramps and other pelvic pain. The diagnosis of endometriosis has been made. The physician has written instructions for this condition. You are instructed to give the patient the printed material and review it with her. How do you approach this patient-teaching opportunity?

_____

_____

_____

_____

_____

5. PREECLAMPSIA (TOXEMIA)

A pregnant patient has been experiencing elevated blood pressure and sudden weight gain. She has been diagnosed with preeclampsia. The physician has printed instructions for this condition. You are instructed to give this information to the patient and her family. How do you approach this patient-teaching opportunity?

_____

_____

_____

_____

_____

6. PLACENT PREVIA

Describe how to teach a patient to prepare for placenta previa.

_____

_____

_____

_____

7. PELVIC INFLAMMATORY DISEASE (PID)

You have been asked to present to a group of high school students on how to prevent PID and STD. Discuss where to obtain the most recent and reliable references, best prevention strategies, and materials to distribute,

_____

_____

_____

_____

Circle the letter of the choice that best completes the statement or answers the question.

1. Treatment of gonorrhea has become more complex because:

   a. Patients with symptoms neglect to seek treatment.

   b. Many strains of *Neisseria gonorrhoeae* have become resistant to antimicrobials.

   c. Many people are allergic to penicillin.

   d. Abstinence from sexual contact is not required once treatment has begun.

2. Genital herpes is not curable, but drug therapy may reduce the frequency and duration of outbreaks. Which medication(s) is(are) frequently used to treat this disease?

   a. Acyclovir (Zovirax)

   b. Famciclovir (Famvir)

   c. Valacyclovir (Valtrex)

   d. All of the above

3. Which of the following statements is(are) associated with the use of sildenafil (Viagra)?

   a. Men who have had a heart attack should not take Viagra.

   b. Viagra may cause temporary vision changes (blurred vision or color changes).

   c. Both of the above are true.

   d. Neither of the above is true.

4. Benign prostatic hyperplasia (BPH) is a common condition of men 50 years and older. Which of the following medications should be avoided with this condition?

   a. Pseudoephedrine (Sudafed)

   b. Doxazosin (Cardura)

   c. Finasteride (Proscar)

   d. Tamsulosin (Flomax)

5. Which of the following may be useful in the treatment of menopause?

   a. Conjugated hormone (Premarin)

   b. Alendronate (Fosamax)

   c. Weight-bearing exercise

   d. All of the above

6. Drug categories for reproductive hormone replacement include:

   a. Androgens.

   b. Estrogens.

   c. Progestins.

   d. All of the above.

ESSAY QUESTION

Write a response to the following question or statement. Use a separate sheet of paper if more space is needed.

1. Discuss the cause, symptoms and signs, and treatment of premature labor.

_____

_____

_____

_____

_____

_____

_____

_____

_____

_____

_____

_____

_____

_____

2. Discuss the prognosis of Paget disease of the breast.

_____

_____

_____

_____

3. Describe the symptoms of prostate cancer.

_____

_____

_____

_____

4. Explain the etiology of the two basic types of ovarian cysts.

_____

_____

_____

_____

5. Describe the difference between primary amenorrhea and primary dysmenorrhea.

_____

_____

_____

_____

6. List contraception options that are considered barrier methods for birth control.

_____

7. List and describe contraception options that are non-barrier methods for birth control.

_____

_____

_____

_____

_____

_____

_____

_____

_____

_____

_____

_____

8. Which methods of birth control are permanent options?

_____

_____

_____

CERTIFICATION EXAMINATION REVIEW

Circle the letter of the choice that best completes the statement or answers the question.

1. Genital warts and many different types of cancer develop from:

   a. Syphilis.

   b. Human papillomavirus (HPV).

   c. Chlamydia.

   d. None of the above.

2. Pelvic inflammatory disease, septicemia, and septic arthritis are complications that may develop from untreated:

   a. Syphilis.

   b. HPV.

   c. Gonorrhea.

   d. None of the above.

3. When functioning endometrial tissue is present outside the uterine cavity, the condition is called:

   a. Septicemia.

   b. Gonorrhea.

   c. Uterine cancer.

   d. None of the above.

4. Dyspareunia is more common in:

   a. Men.

   b. Women.

   c. Teenagers.

   d. Toddlers.

5. Impotence may be caused from:

   a. Use of recreational drugs.

   b. Use of hypertensive medications.

   c. Drinking alcohol.

   d. All of the above.

6. Protrusion of the rectum into the bladder is a:

   a. Cystocele.

   b. Rectal fissure.

   c. Rectocele.

   d. None of the above.

7. Pain that occurs at ovulation is called:

   a. Premenstrual syndrome.

   b. Mittelschmerz.

   c. Both a and b.

   d. None of the above.

8. A Pap smear may be a valuable tool in diagnosing:

   a. Cervical cancer.

   b. Breast cancer.

   c. Testicular cancer.

   d. All of the above.

9. Herpes simplex virus:

   a. Is not curable.

   b. Is easily treated.

   b. Is only detected by a Pap smear.

   b. None of the above.

10. A digital rectal examination, blood test for prostate-specific antigen (PSA), and biopsy to confirm are all evaluations for:

    a. Prostate cancer.

    b. Testicular cancer.

    c. Bladder cancer.

    d. None of the above.

11. Signs of hyperemesis gravidarum may include:

    a. Dehydration.

    b. Abnormal urinalysis.

    c. Abnormal blood chemistries.

    d. All of the above.

12. Premenstrual dysphoric disorder (PMDD) refers to:

    a. Toxemia.

    b. Chlamydia.

    c. Morning sickness.

    d. Severe premenstrual syndrome (PMS).

218

13. The HPV vaccine is:

    a. A major advance in the prevention of cervical cancer.

    b. Recommended in certain age groups for girls, women, and men.

    c. Given as three doses.

    d. All of the above.

14. 4-D Ultrasound:

    a. Adds time as a fourth dimension.

    b. Is only useful to image the unborn.

    c. Results in live images of the unborn child.

    d. Both a and c.

15. Which statement is NOT true about diseases of the breast?

    a. Changes in the breast tissue such as lumps or nipple crusting are not concerns for investigation.

    b. Men do experience diseases of the breast.

    c. Diseases of the breast range from mild to fatal.

    d. The vast majority of breast diseases are diagnosed through abnormal mammogram findings.

16. The most reliable screening method for detecting a tumor of the testicle is:

    a. Monthly testicular self-examination.

    b. Biopsy.

    c. MRI.

    d. The PSA blood test.

17. The most commonly reported notifiable disease in the United States is:

    a. Vaginitis.

    b. Endometriosis.

    c. Chlamydia.

    d. Gonorrhea.

18. The modes of transmission of Hepatitis B include:

    a. Contact with blood, semen, or vaginal secretions.

    b. Sharing contaminated needles or accidental inoculation.

    c. From an infected mother to her infant during birth.

    d. All of the above.

19. Peritonitis is:

    a. A condition that requires prompt and aggressive medical intervention.

    b. Also referred to as cholecystitis.

    c. Caused by short bowel syndrome.

    d. None of the above.

20. The most common male sexual disorder is:

    a. Torsion of the testicle.

    b. Erectile dysfunction (ED)/impotence.

    c. Infertility.

    d. Orchitis.

21. The two greatest risk factors for breast cancer in women are:

    a. Increased age and female gender.

    b. Poor diet and lack of exercise.

    c. Smoking and/or excessive alcohol intake.

    d. Hormonal and genetic factors.

22. In postmenopausal women, what symptom should prompt evaluation for malignancy?

    a. Cystocele

    b. Lack of uterine bleeding

    c. Any uterine bleeding

    d. None of the above

23. Which statements are true about prostate cancer?

    a. It rarely occurs before age 40.

    b. It occurs much more commonly in black men.

    c. Annual screening usually begins at age 50.

    d. All of the above are true.

24. The incidence of STDs is increasing among:

    a. Senior citizens.

    b. Men having sex with men (MSM).

    c. Women.

    d. Both b and c.

25. The most common gynecologic malignancy is:

    a. Endometrial cancer.

    b. Vaginal cancer.

    c. Ovarian cancer.

    d. Vulvar cancer.

26. What STD has an prolonged incubation period of 1 to 6 months?

    a. Gonorrhea

    b. Trichomoniasis

    c. Genetal herpes

    d. Genital warts

27. STDs are a public health problem that require state reporting (vary from state to state). However, several STDs *must* be reported. Which of the following agencies must STDs be reported to?

    a. BCB

    b. MSM

    c. CDC

    d. PID

28. What is the cause of toxic shock syndrome?

    a. Changes in the ovarian production of certain hormones.

    b. Fungal infections are the most common cause.

    c. Retrograde menstruation is believed to be the most likely cause.

    d. The cause is thought to be an increase in staphylococcal colonization on superabsorbent tampons.

Scenario

A young patient is in the office after the patient's first sexual encounter without the use of any protection. The patient is now concerned about contracting a STD or even getting pregnant. Upon further information gathering, it becomes known the sexual partner has had previous sexual encounters and is bisexual. The young patient is worried and needs guidance.

QUESTION:

How do you reassure and explain what to expect during the physician's examination? Discuss what will happen during the exam. Research the internet for known treatments.

Chapter **12** **Diseases and Conditions of the Reproductive System**

13 Neurologic Diseases and Conditions

WORD DEFINITIONS

Define the following basic medical terms.

1. Bradycardia _____

2. Cephalgia _____

3. Craniotomy _____

4. Dilated _____

5. Dysarthric _____

6. Empyema _____

7. Flaccid _____

8. Hemicranial _____

9. Hemiparesis _____

10. Hypotension _____

11. Intervertebral _____

12. Intracranial _____

13. Laminectomy _____

14. Photophobia _____

15. Sequela _____

16. Syncope _____

17. Aphasia _____

18. Aura _____

19. Cephalalgia _____

20. Contrecoup _____

21. Craniotomy _____

22. Epidural   _____

23. Hematoma   _____

24. Hemiplegia   _____

25. Paraplegia   _____

GLOSSARY TERMS

Define the following chapter glossary terms.

1. Autosomal   _____

2. Cauterize   _____

3. Demyelination   _____

4. Diplopia   _____

5. Encephalitis   _____

6. Ergot   _____

7. Fibrin   _____

8. Foramen   _____

9. Hemiparesis   _____

10. Intractable   _____

11. Lumbar puncture   _____

12. Neurotransmitter   _____

13. Nuchal rigidity   _____

14. Paresis   _____

15. Plasmapheresis   _____

SHORT ANSWER

Answer the following questions.

1. Identify the difference between efferent and afferent nerves.

_____

_____

2. Identify the cause of cerebrovascular accidents.

_____

_____

3. Cite another name for a transient ischemic attack (TIA).

_____

4. List some symptoms of a TIA.

_____

5. Which is more serious, a concussion or a cerebral contusion?

_____

6. Identify the common complication of a depressed skull fracture.

_____

_____

7. Identify the most frequent cause of a depressed skull.

_____

_____

8. What is the goal of treatment for spinal cord injuries?

_____

_____

9. List the symptoms of degenerative disk disease.

_____

_____

_____

10. Name the function of an intervertebral disk.

_____

11. List causes of sciatic nerve injury.

_____

225

12. List tests used to diagnose epilepsy.

_____

13. Identify the types of medications that are used to treat epilepsy.

_____

14. Encephalitis is usually the result of a bite from which insect?

_____

15. List possible treatments for a brain abscess.

_____

16. Explain why a lumbar puncture is contraindicated if the patient has a brain abscess.

_____

17. Identify the symptoms of Guillain-Barré syndrome.

_____

_____

18. Identify the vaccines that have helped eliminate cases of poliomyelitis.

_____

19. Cite the statistics for overall 5-year survival of all types of brain tumors.

_____

20. Identify the area of the skull involved with a basilar skull fracture.

_____

21. Which physical manifestations alert the physician to order images of the cranial vault to investigate for a basilar skull fracture?

_____

22. Name the possible routes through which the poliomyelitis virus may enter the body.

_____

23. How are primary brain tumors classified?

_____

24. Identify the race having the highest incidence of brain tumors.

_____

25. How are the cranial nerves assessed during a neurologic examination?

_____

26. Referring to Figure 13-3, *C*, how many pairs of cervical nerves are there? How many pairs of lumbar nerves?

_____

27. List signs of early meningitis.

_____

28. Explain the difference between a closed and an open head injury. List examples. Refer to the text.

_____

29. Referring to text and the Evolve website *E13-11*, identify the types of seizures that may occur.

_____

30. Explain status epilepticus.

_____

FILL IN THE BLANKS

Fill in the blanks with the correct terms. A word list has been provided. Words used twice are indicated with a (2).

Word List
12, blow, brain, breathing, bruising, cartilage, central, chewing, depressed, entire, epilepsy, frontal, head, impact, intervention, life threatening, localized, lower extremities, medulla oblongata, migraine, neurons, occipital, peripheral, spinal cord (2), spine, swallowing, temporal, violent

1. Electrical impulses are carried throughout the body by _____.

2. The two divisions of the nervous system are the _____ nervous system and the _____ nervous system.

3. The central nervous system (CNS) includes the _____ and _____ _____.

4. Five pairs of the cranial nerves originate in the _____, an extension of the spinal cord.

5. The _____ is divided into 31 segments.

6. A cerebral concussion is a(an) _____ of the cerebral tissue that is caused by _____ back-and-forth movement of the head as in an acceleration-deceleration insult.

7. A contusion of the brain is caused by a(an) _____ to the _____ or a(an) _____ against a hard surface, as in an automobile accident.

8. When a portion of the skull is broken and pushed in on the brain, causing injury, it is said to be a(an) _____ skull fracture.

9. Paraplegia results in paralysis of the _____ and usually the trunk.

10. Intervertebral disks are soft pads of _____ located between the vertebrae that make up the _____.

11. Headaches may be acute or chronic and located in the _____, _____, or _____ regions of the head.

12. Before the onset of a headache, many persons who experience _____ headaches have visual auras.

13. Partial seizures do not involve the _____ brain but arise from a _____ _____ area in the brain.

14. Anticonvulsant medications are the treatment of choice for _____.

15. Patients with amyotrophic lateral sclerosis (ALS) have difficulty with speech, _____, _____, and _____ and eventually require a ventilator.

16. Status epilepticus is a _____ event. Immediate _____ may afford a positive outcome.

ANATOMIC STRUCTURES

Identify the structures in the following anatomic diagrams. For number 8, identify the type of paralysis that each illustration represents.

1. The normal brain

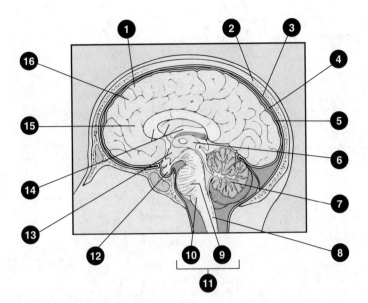

(1) _____

(2) _____

(3) _____

(4) _____

(5) _____

(6) _____

(7) _____

(8) _____

(9) _____

(10) _____

(11) _____

(12) _____

(13) _____

(14) _____

(15) _____

(16) _____

2. The spinal cord

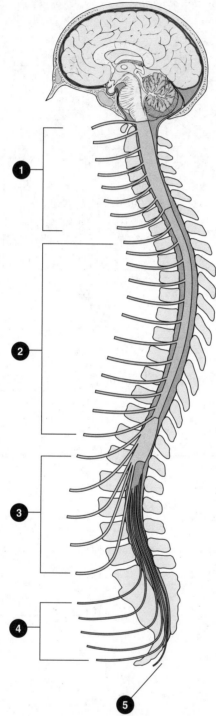

(1) _____

(2) _____

(3) _____

(4) _____

(5) _____

3. The neuron

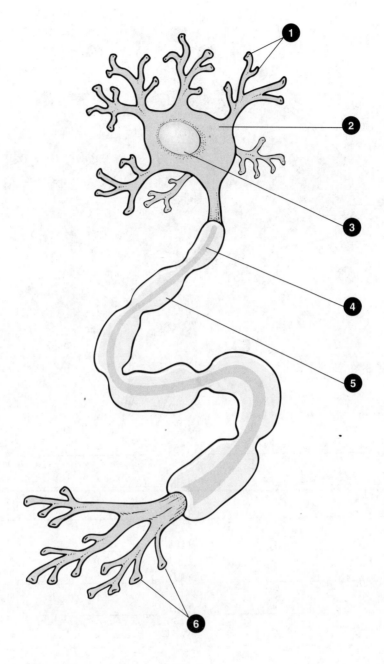

(1) _____

(2) _____

(3) _____

(4) _____

(5) _____

(6) _____

4. Functional areas of the brain

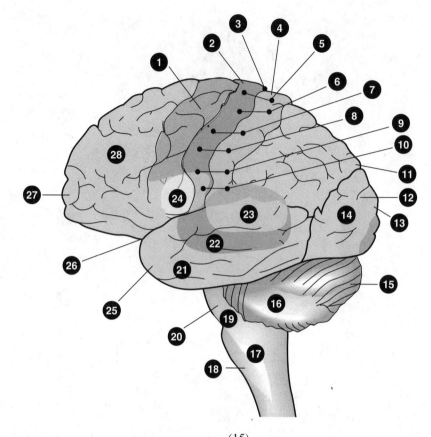

(1) _____   (15) _____

(2) _____   (16) _____

(3) _____   (17) _____

(4) _____   (18) _____

(5) _____   (19) _____

(6) _____   (20) _____

(7) _____   (21) _____

(8) _____   (22) _____

(9) _____   (23) _____

(10) _____   (24) _____

(11) _____   (25) _____

(12) _____   (26) _____

(13) _____   (27) _____

(14) _____   (28) _____

5. The peripheral nervous system

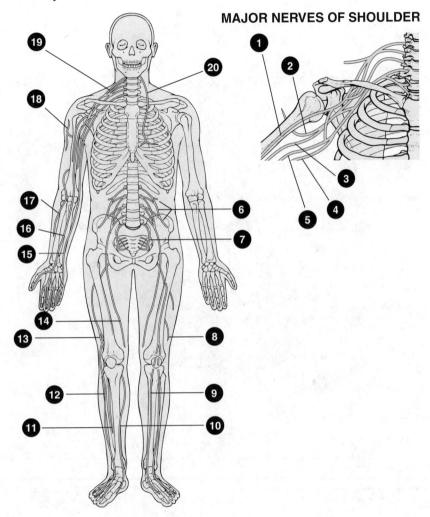

MAJOR NERVES OF SHOULDER

(1) _____	(11) _____
(2) _____	(12) _____
(3) _____	(13) _____
(4) _____	(14) _____
(5) _____	(15) _____
(6) _____	(16) _____
(7) _____	(17) _____
(8) _____	(18) _____
(9) _____	(19) _____
(10) _____	(20) _____

6. The cranial nerves

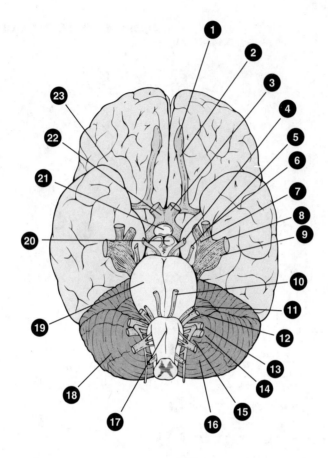

(1) _____   (13) _____

(2) _____   (14) _____

(3) _____   (15) _____

(4) _____   (16) _____

(5) _____   (17) _____

(6) _____   (18) _____

(7) _____   (19) _____

(8) _____   (20) _____

(9) _____   (21) _____

(10) _____   (22) _____

(11) _____   (23) _____

(12) _____

7. Major arteries of the head and neck

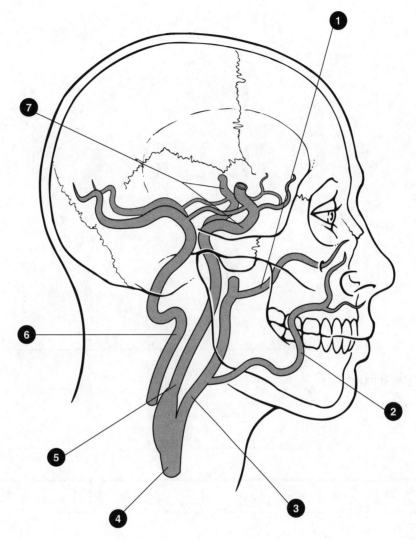

(1) _____

(2) _____

(3) _____

(4) _____

(5) _____

(6) _____

(7) _____

8. Types of paralysis

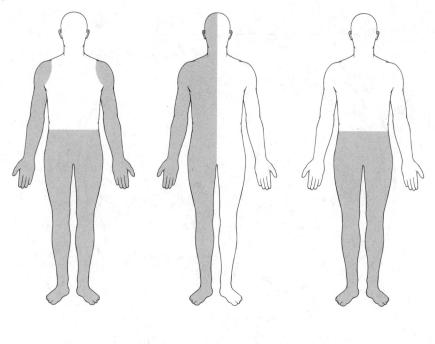

_____ _____ _____

9. Identify the functional components of the nervous system.

(1) _____

(2) _____

(3) _____

(4) _____

PATIENT SCREENING

For each of the following scenarios, explain how and why you would schedule an appointment or suggest a referral based on the patient's reported symptoms. First review the "Guidelines for Patient-Screening Exercises" found on p. iv in the Introduction.

1. A patient's wife calls to report that her husband is experiencing weakness and numbness down one side of the body, dizziness, and confusion. He is conscious. How do you respond to this call?

_____

_____

_____

_____

2. The mother of a 12-year-old boy calls the office and tells you that her son fell down the stairs and experienced an immediate loss of consciousness. This episode lasted for approximately 5 minutes. He has regained consciousness and is experiencing a headache, nausea, vomiting, blurred vision, and photophobia (sensitivity to light). He also is irritable. How do you handle this call?

_____

_____

_____

_____

3. A female patient calls advising that she is having pain that radiates down her back, hip, and leg. She describes the pain as burning and constant, accompanied by the slight loss of motor function in the leg. How do you respond to this call?

_____

_____

_____

_____

4. A female patient calls the office to report that she is experiencing severe head pain. She has a history of migraine headaches. She also is seeing flashing lights and is very sensitive to light. She tells you that she must have something for the terrible pain. She also complains of nausea. How do you respond to this call?

_____

_____

_____

_____

5. A patient's wife calls the office saying that her husband has experienced a sudden onset of memory loss, primarily concerning current and present events. He asks her repetitive questions such as, "Where are we going?" "Why are we going there?" "Where am I?" and "Why did we do that?" He appears confused but knows who and where he is. How do you handle this call?

_____

_____

_____

_____

6. A mother calls the office stating that her 8-year-old son has come home from school early. She says he is complaining of a severe headache that started suddenly about an hour ago. He is nauseated and has started to vomit. She says he refuses to turn his head from side to side and that his eyes keep looking to the left. How would you handle this call?

_____

_____

_____

_____

237

7. A man calls the office stating that his wife just woke up and has a funny feeling in the left side of her face. She cannot smile or close her left eye. She says she cannot taste anything. She is complaining of pain behind her left ear radiating around to her face. She is drooling. How would you handle this call?

_____

_____

_____

_____

PATIENT TEACHING

For each of the following scenarios, outline the appropriate patient teaching you would perform. First review the "Guidelines for Patient-Teaching Exercises" found on p. iv in the Introduction.

1. CEREBROVASCULAR ACCIDENT (CVA) AND TRANSIENT ISCHEMIC ATTACK (TIA)
   These patients usually have been seen in an emergency facility and have come to the office for follow-up care. The physician has printed information regarding both conditions and comparison of the conditions. You are asked to give this information to a patient and family who have experienced CVA or TIA. How do you approach this patient-teaching opportunity?

_____

_____

_____

_____

_____

_____

2. HEAD INJURY
   A patient has experienced a traumatic insult to the head. He has been released from the emergency facility and is in the office for follow-up care. The physician has printed material about closed head injuries. You are instructed by the physician to give this information to the patient and family members. How do you proceed with this patient-teaching opportunity?

_____

_____

_____

_____

_____

_____

3. Ruptured Disk

A patient has been experiencing severe lower back pain. A diagnosis of ruptured lumbar disk has been made. You are instructed by the physician to give printed information to the patient. How do you handle this patient-teaching opportunity?

_____

_____

_____

_____

_____

_____

4. Migraine Headache

A patient has been diagnosed with a migraine headache. The physician has printed instructions for therapy for this condition. You have been instructed to review these instructions with the patient and give her a copy of the information. How do you handle this patient-teaching opportunity?

_____

_____

_____

_____

_____

_____

5. Parkinson's Disease

A patient was recently diagnosed with Parkinson's disease. The physician has written instructions and information concerning this condition. The physician asks you to give the printed information to the patient and family and review it with them. How do you handle this patient-teaching opportunity?

_____

_____

_____

_____

_____

_____

6. SEIZURE ACTIVITY

A patient was recently diagnosed with partial complex seizures. The physician has written instructions and information concerning this condition. The physician asks you to give the printed information to the patient and family and review it with them. How do you handle this patient-teaching opportunity?

_____

_____

_____

_____

_____

_____

_____

PHARMACOLOGY QUESTIONS

Circle the letter of the choice that best completes the statement or answers the question.

1. Treatment of stroke may include which of the following medications?

   a. Aspirin

   b. Metaproterenol (Lopressor)

   c. Lisinopril (Zestril)

   d. Diazepam (Valium)

2. Migraine headaches have been treated with many different types of therapy. Which of the following is not a common therapy of migraine treatment?

   a. Sumatriptan (Imitrex)

   b. Propranolol (Inderal)

   c. Dipyridamole (Persantine)

   d. Ibuprofen (Motrin)

3. Which of the following is not considered a medication for the treatment of epilepsy?

   a. Phenobarbital

   b. Valproic acid (Depakote)

   c. Phenytoin (Dilantin)

   d. Gemfibrozil (Lopid)

4. Which of the following drug combinations is frequently used in the treatment of Parkinson's disease?

   a. Phenytoin/phenobarbital

   b. Carbidopa/levodopa (Sinemet)

   c. Diazepam/lorazepam (Valium and Ativan)

   d. Atenolol/hydrochlorothiazide (Tenormin and Hydrodiuril)

ESSAY QUESTIONS

Write a response to the following questions or statements. Use a separate sheet of paper if more space is needed.

1. Compare and contrast subdural and epidural hematomas.

_____

_____

_____

_____

_____

_____

_____

_____

_____

_____

_____

2. When is a neurologic assessment appropriate?

_____

_____

_____

_____

3. Describe the cause of a herniated and bulging disk.

_____

_____

_____

_____

_____

4. Discuss the cause of TIA.

_____

_____

_____

_____

5. What is the function of the *Circle of Willis*?

_____

_____

_____

_____

6. What are the preventative measures for vascular disorders?

_____

_____

_____

_____

CERTIFICATION EXAMINATION REVIEW

Circle the letter of the choice that best completes the statement or answers the question.

1. Efferent nerves transmit impulses:

    a. Away from the brain and spinal cord.

    b. Toward the brain and spinal cord.

    c. Both a and b.

    d. Neither a nor b.

2. Afferent nerves:

    a. Transmit impulses away from the brain and spinal cord.

    b. Transmit impulses toward the brain and spinal cord.

    c. Are motor nerves.

    d. Both a and c.

3. Chronic alcohol intoxication, toxicity, and infectious disease are possible causes of:

    a. Neuroblastoma.

    b. Trigeminal neuralgia.

    c. Peripheral neuritis.

    d. Guillain-Barré syndrome.

4. A TIA is a _____ episode of impaired neurologic functioning caused by a lack of blood flow to a portion of the brain.

a. Permanent

b. Chronic

c. Temporary

d. Persistent

5. Paraplegia is paralysis that involves loss of motor and sensory control of the trunk and:

a. One extremity.

b. Two extremities.

c. Four extremities.

d. No extremities.

6. Pill-rolling tremor of thumb and forefinger, muscular rigidity, masklike facial expression, and shuffling gait are all signs of:

a. Bell's palsy.

b. Parkinson's disease.

c. Epilepsy.

d. Neuropathy.

7. The blood, penetrating trauma, and infection in adjoining structures such as the ear or sinuses are all routes in which infectious organisms:

a. May reach the brain and cause infection.

b. May reach the brain and cause a stroke.

c. May reach the brain and cause a subdural hematoma.

d. May reach the brain and cause restless leg syndrome.

8. Meningitis is an inflammation of the:

a. Brain.

b. Spinal cord.

c. Membranes covering the brain and spinal cord.

d. Both a and b.

9. Poliomyelitis:

a. Is not diagnosed as frequently as it was before 1960.

b. Is a highly contagious viral disease that affects the anterior horn cells of the gray matter in the spinal cord.

c. Is a bacterial disease.

d. Both a and b.

10. The prognosis for patients with tumors involving the brain is:

a. Poor.

b. Always death.

243

    c. Good.

    d. Difficult to project.

11. Migraine headaches:

    a. Are periodic.

    b. Are sometimes incapacitating.

    c. May be triggered by certain foods in some patients.

    d. All of the above.

12. Hemiparesis is a paralysis involving:

    a. One extremity.

    b. Four extremities.

    c. Either half of the body.

    d. No paralysis.

13. Huntington's chorea is:

    a. A disorder caused by an infection.

    b. An inherited disorder.

    c. Characterized by dancelike movements.

    d. Both b and c.

14. Amyotrophic lateral sclerosis causes symptoms of:

    a. Pill rolling and shuffling of feet.

    b. Progressive destruction of motor neurons, resulting in muscle atrophy.

    c. Dancelike movements and a decline in mental function.

    d. Paralysis.

15. What is the cause of RLS?

    a. Stress

    b. Emotional events

    c. Alcohol intoxication

    d. The exact cause is unknown.

16. When a patient experienced a loss of consciousness, as being 'knocked out.' This is a sign of which injury?

    a. Cerebral contusion

    b. Cerebral concussion

    c. Depressed skull fracture

    d. Spinal cord injury

Scenario

A healthy young male patient age 17 years was involved in a car accident and lost consciousness. While in the medical facility, the patient regained consciousness and is complaining of a headache, shoulder and back pain. The patient's legal guardian was contacted and is very worried and anxious; the 17-year-old has never been previously sick or injuried.

QUESTIONS:

1. Identify and describe the necessary protocol for treating the three different types of concussions. Use the internet to research the known treatments.

   _____

   _____

   _____

   _____

   _____

2. What protocol does the medical staff take in dealing with the worried legal guardian?

   _____

   _____

   _____

   _____

   _____

14 Mental Disorders

WORD DEFINITIONS

Define the following basic medical terms.

1. Aberration   _____

2. Affect   _____

3. Cognitive   _____

4. Detoxification   _____

5. Deficit   _____

6. Delusion   _____

7. Febrile   _____

8. Genitourinary   _____

9. Intermittent   _____

10. Intramuscular   _____

11. Lethargy   _____

12. MRI   _____

13. Musculoskeletal   _____

14. Narcissistic   _____

15. Neurochemical   _____

16. Neurotic   _____

17. Neurotransmitters   _____

18. Paranoid   _____

19. Postulated   _____

20. Precipitate   _____

21. Psychological pain   _____

22. Psychotic   _____

23. Spontaneously   _____

24. Amyloid   _____

25. Circadian rhythm   _____

26. Deficit   _____

27. Endarterectomy   _____

28. Hypoxia   _____

29. Schizoid   _____

GLOSSARY TERMS

Define the following chapter glossary terms.

1. Amnesia   _____

2. Amyloid   _____

3. Anxiolytic   _____

4. Aphonia   _____

5. Catatonic posturing   _____

6. Continuous positive airway pressure   _____

7. Hallucination   _____

8. Hyperesthesia   _____

9. Mutism   _____

10. Paresthesia   _____

11. Positron emission tomography (PET)   _____

12. Prodromal   _____

13. Pseudoneurologic   _____

14. Psychosis   _____

15. Ventricular shift   _____

SHORT ANSWER

Answer the following questions.

1. Name the anxiety disorder that is caused from an overwhelmingly painful external event.

_____

_____

2. Identify the progressive degenerative disease of the brain in which there is a typical profile in the loss of mental and physical functioning. (It is the most frequent cause of deterioration of intellectual capacity or dementia.)

_____

3. List some causes of mental illness.

_____

4. List the criteria for diagnosing intellectual developmental disorder.

_____

_____

5. What is the cure for intellectual developmental disorder?

_____

6. Chronic anxiety that is inappropriate can develop into what type of disorder?

_____

7. Dementia involves deterioration of which three functions?

_____

8. Identify the disorder that is characterized by intense mood swings from manic to depressive.

_____

9. Identify the drug of choice used during an acute manic phase of bipolar disease.

_____

10. When are most learning disorders in children first identified?

_____

11. Identify a major factor that creates and maintains stuttering.

_____

12. List the five types of pervasive development disorders as identified in the autistic spectrum.

_____

13. List the three subtypes identified in attention-deficit hyperactivity disorder.

_____

_____

14. Describe oppositional defiant disorder.

_____

15. Name the medication used to treat Tourette's syndrome.

_____

16. What four symptoms are nearly always present when a child has autism?

_____

_____

17. List examples of simple motor tics.

_____

18. List causes of dementia.

_____

_____

19. Explain hallucination.

_____

20. List the four major groups of drugs that are often abused.

_____

21. Describe bipolar disorder.

_____

22. Describe major depressive disorder.

_____

23. List the phases of the grief process as identified by Elisabeth Kübler-Ross.

_____

24. Anxiety disorders include four specific anxiety disorders. List these disorders.

_____

25. Identify the disorder in which the anxiety that a patient experiences is converted to a physical or somatic symptom as a defense mechanism.

_____

26. Name the associative subtypes of pain disorders.

_____

27. Identify the type of preoccupation that a patient suffering from hypochondriasis experiences.

_____

28. A patient who is fully aware that he or she is not sick or ill but seeks medical attention anyway would be having symptoms of which condition?

_____

29. Do somatoform disorders include a group of mental disorders in which physical symptoms have an organic cause?

_____

30. Identify the test that is used to assess sleep disorders.

_____

31. To be diagnosed with insomnia, how long must sleeplessness endure?

_____

32. Identify the group of sleep disorders that includes sleepwalking, night terrors, and nightmares.

_____

33. At what blood alcohol level would a person exhibit the following effects: impairment in coordination, judgment, memory, and comprehension? (Hint: In some states the person would be considered legally drunk.)

_____

34. Identify the phobia associated with a fear of blood.

_____

35. Name the phobia associated with a fear of disease.

_____

36. A person with a narcissistic personality would demonstrate what type of behavior?

_____

37. Which accepted reference offers guidelines for criteria to be used in the clinical setting when diagnosing a mental disorder?

_____

38. What is involved in the treatment of vascular dementia?

_____

39. What is the prognosis for the individual suffering from dementia caused by head trauma?

_____

40. Describe learning disorders.

_____

FILL IN THE BLANKS

Fill in the blanks with the correct terms. A word list has been provided. Words used twice are indicated with a (2).

Word List

acute, adolescence, antidepressants, axis, children (2), contributing factor, cope, counseling, developmental disability, different, differently, difficulty, electroconvulsive, examinations, fear, genetic, hopeless, inability, influence, injectable, intense, Intellectual developmental disorder, linked, mathematics, medical, modern, Naltrexone not, numerous causes, pain, pleasure, preschool routine, prevention, psychotropic drugs, reading, real, skill, social, stimulants, vivitrol, writing

1. Stress is considered a _____ of mental disorders.

2. Mental illness has been _____ to the patient's _____ to _____ with stress imposed by _____ society.

3. Psychological pain is _____ and _____ and can _____ physical health.

4. Modern therapeutic approaches include control of symptoms with _____ _____, including antipsychotic drugs, _____, anxiolytics, CNS _____, and antimanic agents; hospitalization during _____ episodes; psychotherapy; and _____ therapy and group therapy.

5. Play therapy is included in _____ for some _____.

6. Mental illnesses are categorized by _____. Each axis represents a _____ part of the diagnosis.

7. Intellectual developmental disorder, _____ _____ _____, is not a disease but a wide range of conditions with many causes.

8. Signs of intellectual developmental disorder may be evident on well-baby _____ or during _____ checkups.

9. Intellectual developmental disorder has _____, many of which are unidentifiable.

10. Learning disabilities occur when _____ learn things _____ in a manner that is _____ normal.

11. The person with learning disorders exhibits _____ in acquiring a _____ in a specific area of learning such as _____, _____, and _____.

12. Schizophrenia is thought to be _____; therefore there is no known _____.

13. Suicide intervention is an attempt by _____, mental health, and community services to assist the depressed individual through the _____ situation.

14. Personality disorders typically begin in _____.

15. Avoidance personality disorder avoids any _____ situation because of _____ of criticism, disapproval, or rejection.

16. Individuals with schizoid personality disorder appear to lack or fail to show emotions of _____ or _____.

17. As of June 2006, _____ _____ became available as an _____ medication, which must be given monthly by a health care professional.

For each of the following scenarios, explain how and why you would schedule an appointment or suggest a referral based on the patient's reported symptoms. First review the "Guidelines for Patient-Screening Exercises" found on p. iv in the Introduction.

1. A father calls the office saying that his 6-year-old son is experiencing a speech pattern of frequent repetitions or prolongations of sounds or syllables. The fluency of his normal speech is punctuated with broken words and word repetitions. How do you respond to this call?

    _____

    _____

    _____

2. The daughter of an older patient calls saying that her father is experiencing loss of short-term memory, the inability to concentrate, impairment of reasoning, and subtle changes in personality. He also is restless, having trouble sleeping, and combative. How do you handle this call?

    _____

    _____

    _____

3. A female patient calls the office stating that she is experiencing deep and persistent sadness, despair, and hopelessness. She says that she is having problems sleeping and does not want to eat. This started a few days ago and is getting worse. She wants help. How do you handle this call?

    _____

    _____

    _____

4. A patient's husband calls the office saying that his wife is having problems sleeping and is irritable. She is having nightmares about a fatal automobile accident she witnessed 3 months ago. She refuses to ride in a car. He is requesting an appointment. How do you handle this call?

    _____

    _____

    _____

    _____

5. A male patient calls the office and tells you that he is having difficulty falling asleep and staying asleep. He also says that he is physically and mentally tired, groggy, tense, irritable, and anxious in the morning. He states that his sleep is not restorative. How do you handle this call?

_____

_____

_____

_____

6. A 45-year-old female patient calls the office asking for an appointment, as she recently has been experiencing what she labels "panic attacks." She says these attacks have started suddenly and that she is experiencing palpitations, has a rapid pulse, and is short of breath during the attacks. She also relates that she gets really sweaty, trembles, and experiences chest pain and dizziness. She says she feels that she is going "crazy." How do you handle this call?

_____

_____

_____

_____

7. A 30-year-old male patient calls the office stating that he is having problems controlling his urge to drink. During the last month he has experienced being arrested for public intoxication, and he states that he cannot go through that again. His job is in jeopardy and he needs help stopping drinking. How do you handle this call?

_____

_____

_____

_____

PATIENT TEACHING

For each of the following scenarios, outline the appropriate patient teaching you would perform. First review the "Guidelines for Patient-Teaching Exercises" found on p. iv in the Introduction.

1. STUTTERING
   The pediatrician has seen a child after he started having episodes of stuttering. The parents have been advised that the child will probably outgrow the stuttering. The pediatrician has printed information about many childhood communication disorders and suggests that you give it to the parents and review it with them. How do you handle this patient-teaching opportunity?

_____

_____

_____

_____

2. DEMENTIA

The family of a patient who has recently been diagnosed with dementia caused by traumatic brain insult has made an appointment to discuss treatment and potential outcome of the insult. The physician has discussed these matters with the family. She has printed information regarding the potential outcome in this type of situation and asks you to review this information with the family and encourage them to ask questions in the future. How do you handle this patient-teaching opportunity?

_____

_____

_____

_____

3. BIPOLAR DISORDER

A patient has just met with the physician for a review of bipolar disorder. The physician has changed the medications prescribed. He provides printed instructions, and you are instructed to review this information with the patient. How do you handle this patient-teaching opportunity?

_____

_____

_____

_____

4. HYPOCHONDRIASIS

A patient has been seen numerous times for complaints with no documented basis. The physician has made a tentative diagnosis of hypochondriasis. Although the physician has printed instructions for managing these patients, she does not believe that it would be in the best interest of the patient to provide him with the printed information at this time. She has reviewed the suggestions with the patient and instructs you to reinforce this information as you accompany him during the sign-out process. How will you handle this patient-teaching opportunity?

_____

_____

_____

_____

5. INSOMNIA

An individual has been experiencing periods of sleeplessness every night for the past 2 weeks. She complains of being extremely tired and having difficulty performing routine daily activities. The physician has printed suggestions for the patient experiencing insomnia. You are instructed to give her these instructions and review them with her. How do you handle this patient-teaching opportunity?

_____

_____

_____

_____

6. POSTPARTUM DEPRESSION

A young, first-time mom has been diagnosed with postpartum depression. She has been experiencing fatigue, changes in her normal appetite, difficulty sleeping, crying episodes, and poor personal hygiene. She has expressed feelings of anger and thoughts of suicide. She appears sad and also appears to lack interest in anything. She fears being alone and expresses thoughts of killing the infant. You have been instructed to print instructions for this condition and to go over them with the family. How would you handle this patient-teaching opportunity?

_____

_____

_____

_____

7. PHOBIAS

A 36-year-old patient calls the office requesting an appointment for help in controlling her phobia about airplanes and flying. Her husband has won a 20-day trip to Europe and wants her to accompany him. The trip is a month away, and she has to tell him if she will go with him by next week. The trip will involve flying to different countries. She wants to go but is afraid to get on an airplane. She says she knows there is no danger but she doesn't know how to get over this fear. How do you handle this call?

_____

_____

_____

_____

PHARMACOLOGY QUESTIONS

Circle the letter of the choice that best completes the statement or answers the question.

1. Which of the following medications is used in the treatment of ADHD?

   a. Methylphenidate (Ritalin)

   b. Amphetamine salts (Adderall)

   c. Dextroamphetamine (Dexedrine)

   d. All of the above

2. Which of the following ADHD medications is not a DSA schedule II substance?

   a. Atomoxetine (Strattera)

   b. Methylphenidate (Ritalin)

   c. Amphetamine salts (Adderall)

   d. Dextroamphetamine (Dexedrine)

3. Which of the following medications is not a common therapy for Alzheimer's?

   a. Donepezil (Aricept)

   b. Paroxetine (Paxil)

   c. Risperidone (Risperdal)

   d. Vitamin K (Mephyton)

4. Of the following drugs of abuse, which would be considered a stimulant?

    a. Alcohol

    b. Marijuana

    c. Ketamine

    d. Cocaine

5. Many different medications have been used in the treatment of schizophrenia. Which of the following drugs could be used?

    a. Olanzapine (Zyprexa)

    b. Haloperidol (Haldol)

    c. Ziprasidone (Geodon)

    d. All of the above

6. Depression is frequently treated with selective serotonin reuptake inhibitors (SSRIs). Which of the following is in this class?

    a. Fluoxetine (Prozac)

    b. Amitriptyline (Elavil)

    c. Nortriptyline (Pamelor)

    d. None of the above

7. Which of the following medications could be used for the treatment of insomnia?

    a. Methylphenidate (Ritalin)

    b. Pregabalin (Lyrica)

    c. Zolpidem (Ambien)

    d. Both b and c

8. A teacher will notice that the child is not at a standard pace. The school system will then test by the child to evaluate for a discrepancy between ability and performance. This is a sign of what disorder?

    a. Communication disorder

    b. Learning disorder

    c. Pervasive development disorder

    d. Autism spectrum disorder

9. What might be a major factor in stuttering?

    a. Anxiety

    b. Phobia

    c. Streptococcus

    d. Head trauma

ESSAY QUESTIONS

Write a response to the following questions or statements. Use a separate sheet of paper if more space is needed.

1. Explain the physical manifestations of tic disorders. Can the person with this type of disorder control the tics?

_____

_____

_____

_____

_____

_____

_____

_____

_____

_____

_____

_____

2. Explain the manifestations of dementia. Discuss the impact of the disease on the patient, the family, and the community.

_____

_____

_____

_____

_____

_____

_____

_____

_____

_____

_____

_____

_____

_____

3. Why does patient teaching need to be very specific for a patient diagnosed with substance-related disorders?

_____

_____

_____

_____

4. Describe the symptoms and signs of oppositional defiant disorder.

_____

_____

_____

_____

_____

5. Discuss the cause of conversion disorder.

_____

_____

_____

_____

6. What is meant by free-floating anxiety?

_____

_____

_____

7. What is the suggested evidence initiating schizophrenia?

_____

_____

_____

_____

8. What are some of the causes that can lead to drug abuse by individuals?

_____

_____

_____

_____

9. Who is most likely to display symptoms and signs of retardation?

_____

_____

_____

_____

_____

_____

_____

_____

CERTIFICATION EXAMINATION REVIEW

Circle the letter of the choice that best completes the statement or answers the question.

1. Anxiety is a major factor that creates and maintains:

   a. Autistic disorder.

   b. Mood disorder.

   c. Stuttering.

   d. All of the above.

2. Autistic disorder involves symptoms of:

   a. Progressive deterioration of mental capacities.

   b. Extreme withdrawal and lack of social interaction.

   c. Anxiety resulting from an external event of an overwhelming painful nature.

   d. None of the above.

3. Haldol is the drug of choice used to treat:

    a. Alzheimer's disease.

    b. Münchausen's syndrome.

    c. Tourette's disorder.

    d. None of the above.

4. Pancreatitis, cirrhosis, and peripheral neuropathy may be the result of:

    a. Prolonged heavy use of alcohol.

    b. Occasional social drinking.

    c. Excessive use of alcohol.

    d. One drink a day.

5. Bipolar disorder causes symptoms of:

    a. Intense mood swings from manic to depressive.

    b. Motor tics coupled with vocal tics.

    c. Loss of concentration, fatigue, and appetite changes.

    d. All of the above.

6. The grief process has five phases. They are, in order:

    a. Anger, depression, denial, bargaining, and acceptance.

    b. Denial, anger, bargaining, depression, and acceptance.

    c. Depression, anger, denial, acceptance, and bargaining.

    d. None of the above.

7. Electroconvulsive therapy, psychotherapy, and antidepressant drug therapy may be used to treat:

    a. Narcolepsy.

    b. Major depressive disorders.

    c. Somatoform disorders.

    d. All of the above.

8. Tourette's disorder is characterized by:

    a. Intense mood swings from manic to depressive.

    b. Decrease in social interaction.

    c. Vocal and motor tics.

    d. A habit of deliberately annoying others.

9. Suicidal thoughts and actions may be brought on by:

    a. Somatoform disorders.

    b. Autism.

    c. Major depression.

    d. None of the above.

Chapter **14** **Mental Disorders**

10. Anxiety, amnesia, and impotence have been associated with:

    a. Prolonged heavy use of alcohol.

    b. Excessive use of alcohol.

    c. Occasional social drinking.

    d. All of the above.

11. Panic, phobic, and obsessive-compulsive disorders are all included in the group of:

    a. Somatoform disorders.

    b. Anxiety disorders.

    c. Personality disorders.

    d. None of the above.

12. Genetic disorders, infection, trauma, poisoning, early alterations in embryonic developmental general medical conditions, prematurity, and hypoxia are all identifiable causes of:

    a. Autism.

    b. Intellectual developmental disorder.

    c. Anxiety disorders.

    d. None of the above.

SCENARIO

A patient complains of not feeling well, overall lack of energy, excessive sleeping, overeating, craving for carbohydrates, and weight gain. The physician examination included asking a serious of questions, blood tests to rule out a variety of metabolic diseases, general physical—all results returned within normal limits with no predominant diseases. The physician begins a screening for depression and learns the patient is extremely active during summer months, while much more inactive and remains indoors during winter months.

QUESTIONS

a. What do you suspect is this patient's diagnosis?

_____

b. What signs leads you to believe this diagnosis?

_____

_____

_____

_____

c. What is the treatment that is usually prescribed?

_____

_____

_____

_____

15 | Disorders and Conditions Resulting From Trauma

WORD DEFINITIONS

Define the following basic medical terms.

1. Abrasion _____

2. Amnesia _____

3. Appendage _____

4. Autograft _____

5. Avulsion _____

6. Axillae _____

7. Cautery _____

8. Coagulation _____

9. Constricted _____

10. Endemic _____

11. Ergonomics _____

12. Hemostasis _____

13. Hyperthermia _____

14. Hypothermia _____

15. Inoculation _____

16. Myalgia _____

17. Occipital _____

18. Phlebotomist _____

19. Prophylaxis _____

20. Vasculitis _____

21. Analgesic _____

22. Antiseptic _____

23. Tendinitis _____

GLOSSARY TERMS

Define the following chapter glossary terms.

1. Abduction _____

2. Anesthetic _____

3. Apnea _____

4. Cataracts _____

5. Corneal ulcers _____

6. Débride _____

7. Electromyography (EMG) _____

8. Emergency Medical Service (EMS) _____

9. Encephalitis _____

10. Ergonomic _____

11. Maculopapular _____

12. Prothrombin time (PT) _____

13. Steri-Strips _____

14. Vectors _____

15. Venom _____

SHORT ANSWER

Answer the following questions.

1. If a patient experiences an open trauma, which type of prophylactic injection is recommended to prevent an infection?

_____

2. Intimate partner violence may also be referred to as what?

_____

_____

3. If a patient calls the office after being bitten by a snake, what steps should you inform him or her not to take?

_____

4. Identify the name of the rule that is used to determine the percentage of body surface area that is affected when a person sustains burn injuries.

_____

5. Identify which persons are at the greatest risk for sunburn.

_____

_____

6. List some symptoms of early-stage hypothermia.

_____

7. Name the areas of the body that are at high risk for frostbite when exposed to extreme cold.

_____

8. Identify one disease that is transmitted by a mosquito.

_____

_____

9. Name three diseases that may be transmitted by ticks to humans.

_____

10. Name the substance that insects inject when they bite a person.

_____

11. What is the incubation time for a person to become ill between the time he or she is bitten by a tick and when he or she begins to show symptoms of Rocky Mountain spotted fever?

_____

12. When an insect stinger is still attached to the skin after an individual has been bitten, explain the best way to remove it.

_____

13. What are the mild symptoms of altitude sickness?

_____

_____

14. List four species of poisonous snakes found in the United States.

_____

_____

15. What is one way to determine whether a poisonous, rather than a non-poisonous, snake has bitten a patient? (Disregard coral snakes.)

_____

16. Identify the type of poisonous snake responsible for the greatest number of snakebites.

_____

17. Name the nerve that is entrapped when a patient has carpal tunnel syndrome.

_____

18. Are tennis players the only people who are diagnosed with tennis elbow?

_____

19. (True or false?) Deep frostbite warming should not begin until professional medical care can be provided.

_____

20. When a person experiences an electrical burn, what two things will be visible on his or her skin?

_____

_____

21. Identify treatment options for carpal tunnel syndrome.

_____

_____

22. What is the health care worker's responsibility in regard to reporting suggested child abuse and neglect?

_____

_____

23. Identify the three symptoms that lead the physician to diagnose a child with shaken baby syndrome.

_____

24. (True or false?) Emotional abuse is easy to identify.

_____

_____

25. Define sexual abuse.

_____

26. Name the most reliable method to determine a child's paternity.

_____

27. List examples of possible sources of danger involving bioterrorism.

_____

28. By what method could the smallpox virus be spread throughout the population?

_____

29. Identify the area of the body that would be affected if there were an outbreak of plague.

_____

30. List clues that may lead to diagnosis of suspected child abuse.

_____

31. What are the two major factors identified as the incidence and continuation of intimate partner abuse or domestic violence?

_____

32. How long must evidence collected during a sexual assault examination be maintained?

_____

33. List the three typical stages of the cycle of abuse in family abuse.

_____

34. Modification of some causes of cumulative trauma may reduce its incidence or exacerbation. List some of these recommendations.

_____

35. Cumulative trauma is a group of muscular conditions that result from repeated motions performed in the curse of daily activities. Explain this condition.

_____

_____

36. Although they are not specific disease entities, traumatic occurrences do include physical and psychological injuries. How did these injuries derive?

_____

FILL IN THE BLANKS

Fill in the blanks with the correct terms. A word list has been provided.

Word List

analgesic, antiseptic, black widow, bleeding, body, brown recluse, bugs, burn centers, cardiac, coagulation, corneal, doxycycline, ears, eyes, fluorescein, foreign, friction, hypothermia, jagged, leading, nose, nuclear family, pain, respiratory, rough, rust, sand, single parent, smooth, stroke, suture, temperature, tetracycline, thermal, tree, young

1. Physical trauma is the _____ cause of death in _____ people in the United States.

2. Abrasions are caused by _____ from a _____ hard surface.

3. Puncture wounds cause _____ and very little _____.

4. The edges of a laceration may be _____ or _____, depending on the object that did the cutting.

5. Anything that enters a portion of the _____ where it does not belong is considered a _____ body. Common sites for these include the _____, the _____, the _____, and any surface area of the body.

6. Common foreign bodies in the eye include _____, _____, dust, _____, hair, small pieces of metal, small pieces of brush, and _____ branches.

7. Staining the eye with _____ to visualize a _____ abrasion will confirm the presence or previous presence of a foreign body.

8. Major burns are referred to _____ for treatment.

9. The treatment for sunburn includes cooling with cool water and spraying with _____ and _____ sprays.

10. Burns are the results of _____ insults to the tissues.

11. Patients who have experienced electrical shock may be in _____ or _____ failure.

12. Heat _____ occurs when the person has a body _____ of 105° F or higher.

13. If a person's core body temperature drops below 95° F, _____ occurs.

14. People with _____, _____, or scorpion bites should be transported to an emergency facility.

15. The antibiotic treatment of choice for Rocky Mountain spotted fever is _____.

16. With lacerations, bleeding should be controlled by either _____ or _____.

17. With the breakdown of the _____ _____ structure and the stresses of being a _____ _____ the additional task of caring for an elderly person can become an overwhelming burden.

ANATOMIC STRUCTURES

Identify the following wound types.

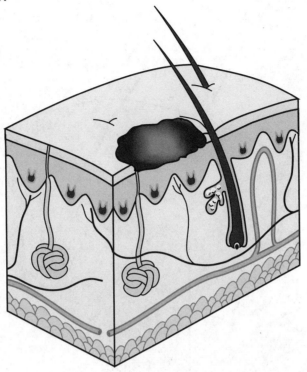

1. _____

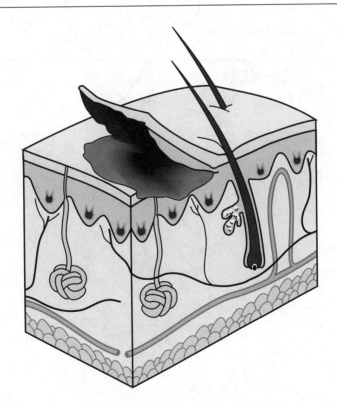

2. _____

Chapter **15** **Disorders and Conditions Resulting From Trauma**

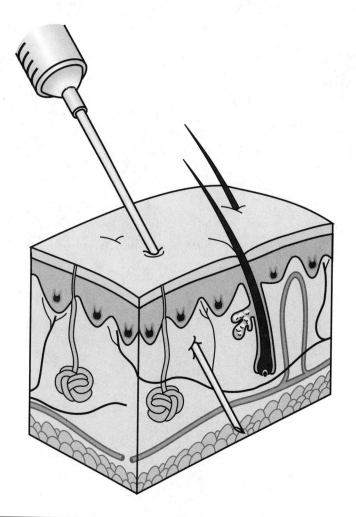

3. _____

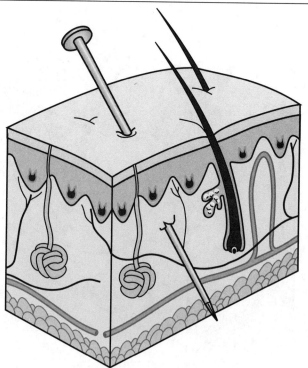

4. _____

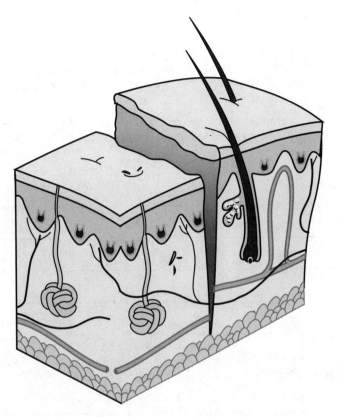

5. _____

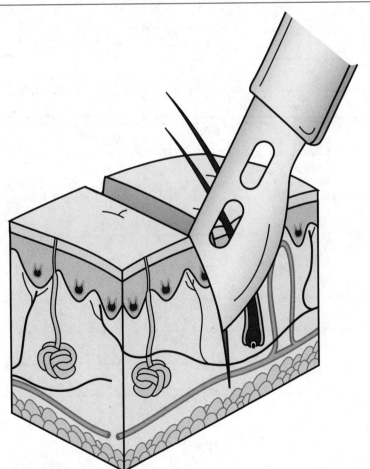

6. _____

PATIENT SCREENING

For each of the following scenarios, explain how and why you would schedule an appointment or suggest a referral based on that patient's reported symptoms. First review the "Guidelines for Patient-Screening Exercises" found on p. iv in the Introduction.

1. A father calls to report that his 4-year-old son has stepped on a nail in a board. The child pulled his foot off the board and nail, and the foot looks red around the site. He wants to know what to do. How do you handle this call?

_____

_____

_____

_____

_____

2. A patient calls the office complaining of feeling stuffiness and something in the ear. He has complaints of pain in the ear canal and decreased hearing capability. How do you respond to this call?

_____

_____

_____

_____

_____

3. A mother calls advising that her 16-year-old son has been out in the extreme cold. She has noticed that the tissue on his face is firm and the skin has a waxy appearance. The skin is very cold to the touch. How do you respond to this call?

_____

_____

_____

_____

_____

4. A female patient calls advising that she is experiencing numbness of hands and fingers with pain in these areas at night. Swelling of the wrist or hand and "fluttering" of the fingers are additional symptoms. How do you handle this call?

_____

_____

_____

_____

_____

_____

5. An older patient calls to tell you that she has noticed bruising on her daughter in various stages of healing and on areas of the body that are concealed by clothing. Her daughter says that she will agree to come to the office. How do you respond?

_____

_____

_____

_____

_____

_____

6. A parent calls and states the 10-year-old son has been playing on the swing set and appears to have what looks like a bite or sting of an insect. The parent requests an appointment with the doctor. How should this call be managed?

_____

_____

_____

_____

_____

PATIENT TEACHING

For each of the following scenarios, outline the appropriate patient teaching you would perform. First review the "Guidelines for Patient-Teaching Exercises" found on p. iv in the Introduction.

1. AVULSION
   A patient has been involved in a traumatic situation experiencing an avulsion to the left hand. After the repair of the involved area is complete, the patient requires instruction on care of the wound. The physician has printed information regarding wound care. You are instructed to give this information to the patient and family and review it. How do you handle this patient-teaching opportunity?

_____

_____

_____

_____

_____

_____

2. FOREIGN BODY IN THE EAR

A parent brought his child in with a small bead in the ear canal that had been in the ear for 2 days. After the physician removed the foreign body, he discussed with the child and parent the problems that may develop when foreign bodies are in a child's ear. You are instructed to provide the parent with printed instructions regarding foreign bodies in the ears, eyes, and nose. How do you handle this patient-teaching opportunity?

_____

_____

_____

_____

_____

_____

3. LIGHTNING STRIKE INJURIES

A patient was struck by lightning a few days ago. He has been released from the hospital and is in the office for a follow-up visit. Having survived the attack, the patient expresses an interest in preventing the situation from occurring again. How do you handle this patient-teaching opportunity?

_____

_____

_____

_____

_____

_____

4. ANIMAL BITES

A parent has brought into the office her child who has recently been bitten by the neighbor's dog. The child was initially treated in an emergency facility and is in the office for a follow-up examination. The parents have received patient-teaching information at the emergency facility, and a report of the incident was made to animal control. The physician asks you to reinforce the printed information given to the parents by the emergency facility. How do you handle this patient-teaching opportunity?

_____

_____

_____

_____

_____

_____

5. CARPAL TUNNEL SYNDROME

A patient comes in complaining of pain to the right hand and wrist along with numbness and tingling in the arm and hand. A diagnosis of carpal tunnel syndrome is made. The physician asks that you review the printed information on carpal tunnel syndrome with the patient. How do you handle this patient-teaching opportunity?

_____

_____

_____

_____

_____

_____

6. PUNTURE WOUND

Describe with the patient the length of time and continued treatment after symptoms abate from puncture wounds.

_____

_____

_____

_____

_____

_____

7. BURN PREVENTION

Patient arrives with multiple burns on arms and legs from a spilled boiling pot of water. Once the physician treats the burns, the order states to teach the patient how to manage the burn care. Discuss the burn care specifics for the patient teaching.

_____

_____

_____

_____

ESSAY QUESTION

Write a response to the following question or statement. Use a separate sheet of paper if more space is needed.
1. Describe the physical indicators that may be present when a child is the victim of child abuse and neglect.

_____

_____

_____

_____

_____

_____

_____

_____

_____

_____

_____

_____

2. What does MRI stand for? Explain how it is beneficial in a puncture wound.

_____

_____

_____

3. Because burn prevention is difficult, discuss the specifics of patient teaching.

_____

_____

_____

_____

Circle the letter of the choice that best completes the statement or answers the question.

1. Victims of abuse can include:

    a. Men.

    b. Women.

    c. Children.

    d. All of the above.

2. Gentle cleansing, approximation and securing of the edges, débridement, suturing, sterile dressing application, and use of tissue glue are all methods to treat a:

    a. Puncture wound.

    b. Laceration.

    c. Burn.

    d. Abrasion.

3. Carpal tunnel syndrome is a repetitive motion injury that involves the _____ nerve.

    a. Sciatic

    b. Median

    c. Brachial plexus

    d. Tibial

4. An avulsion is a soft tissue injury in which:

    a. The outer layer of the skin has been scraped away.

    b. Skin, tissue, and bone are being pulled away from the body.

    c. The wound has a straight, neat edge.

    d. A pointed or sharp object penetrates the soft tissue.

5. An abrasion is a soft tissue injury in which:

    a. The outer layer of the skin has been scraped away.

    b. Skin, tissue, and bone are being pulled away from the body.

    c. The wound has a straight, neat edge.

    d. A pointed or sharp object penetrates the soft tissue.

6. Heat stroke causes symptoms of red, hot, dry skin; headache; dizziness; shortness of breath; and a body temperature of:

    a. 100° to 102° F.

    b. 103° F.

    c. More than 105° F.

    d. 99° F.

7. Thoracic outlet syndrome involves compression of the _____ nerve.

   a. Sciatic

   b. Median

   c. Brachial plexus

   d. Tibial

8. The percentage area of the body burned is determined by using the rule of:

   a. Eights.

   b. Nines.

   c. Tens.

   d. Twenties.

9. Bugs, insects, cereal, peas, beans, grapes, pebbles, and cotton are all foreign bodies sometimes found in a patient's:

   a. Ears.

   b. Eyes.

   c. Eyes and ears.

   d. None of the above.

10. Treatment of frostbite includes:

    a. Vigorous massage of the affected area.

    b. Immersion of the affected part in hot water.

    c. Deep rewarming supervision by health care professionals.

    d. Rubbing with ice.

11. State laws vary, but most require reporting of suggested child abuse and neglect:

    a. By all people.

    b. By health care workers.

    c. By teachers.

    d. Both b and c.

12. Treatment of a puncture wound includes:

    a. Brisk scrubbing of the area with a brush.

    b. Copious irrigation of the wound.

    c. Approximation of the wound edges for suturing.

    d. All of the above.

13. A burn that involves destruction of the skin and underlying tissue is termed:

    a. Superficial.

    b. Partial thickness.

    c. Full thickness.

    d. Radiation.

278

14. In electrical shock, the current:

    a. Follows the path of least resistance.

    b. Always enters the heart.

    c. Destroys the brain tissue.

    d. Does none of the above.

15. The person suffering from hypothermia experiences:

    a. Shivering.

    b. Disorientation.

    c. Fatigue.

    d. All of the above.

16. Tetanus toxoid prophylaxis is important in any person who has sustained open trauma because:

    a. Boosters are required throughout life.

    b. Tetanus toxoid is a broad-spectrum antibiotic.

    c. Organisms that cause tetanus enter the body directly into the bloodstream through wounds.

    d. There is no danger of tetanus being a fatal disorder.

17. Treatment of snakebite includes:

    a. Keeping the victim quiet and transporting him or her to an emergency facility.

    b. Putting a tourniquet around the limb.

    c. Applying ice.

    d. Cutting the wound.

18. Cumulative trauma disorders include:

    a. Carpal tunnel syndrome.

    b. White finger.

    c. Synovitis.

    d. All of the above.

19. Nausea, vomiting, and diarrhea; redness and blistering of skin burns; dehydration; weakness, fatigue, exhaustion, and fainting; hair loss, ulceration of oral mucosa, esophagus, and gastrointestinal (GI) tract; vomiting blood and experiencing bloody stools; bruising; sloughing of the skin; and bleeding from nose, mouth, and gums are symptoms of:

    a. Ingested poison.

    b. Radiation poisoning.

    c. Lightning strike.

    d. Poisonous snakebite.

20. Complications of survivors of lightning strikes include:

    a. Cataracts.

    b. Cervical spine injuries.

c. Ruptured tympanic membranes.

d. All of the above.

21. If an insect stinger is still present and must be removed, what could be the outcome of using forceps or tweezers to remove it?

    a. It takes a long time to sterilize forceps or tweezers.

    b. The use of forceps or tweezers squeezes more venom into the site.

    c. Stingers can be too large for forceps or tweezers.

    d. All of the above.

Scenario #1

A patient was using a chainsaw while using precautions, wore ear plugs, safety glasses, and gloves. When the patient had completed sawing, removal of the ear plugs, safety glasses, and gloves took place. The patient had some facial saw dust and attempted to remove the dust by using a bare hand and brushing away the dust. However, the patient's right eye started blinking and watering. Then the patient rubbed the eye and immediately the eye turned blood shot with intense pain. The patient determined a trip the urgent care was necessary and had a family member take them for care.

QUESTIONS:

1. What is the treatment for a foreign body in the eye?

_____

_____

_____

_____

Scenario #2

A patient was playing baseball and was running to first base when suddenly has severe pain in the back part of the leg and can hardly walk. Patient immediately seeks medical attention, and physician diagnoses the problem as hamstring strain. Physician orders include applying an ACE bandage to the leg.

    The patient has many unanswered questions that were not addressed to the physician. While you are applying the ACE bandage, how will the following questions be answered?

QUESTIONS:

a. Why does the doctor what an ACE bandage apply to his leg?

_____

_____

_____

_____

b. How should I treat a hamstring strain?

_____

_____

_____

_____

c. What is the difference between a strain and a sprain?

_____

_____

_____

_____